WHO Technical Report Series
894

OBESITY: PREVENTING AND MANAGING THE GLOBAL EPIDEMIC

I0616533

Report of a
WHO Consultation

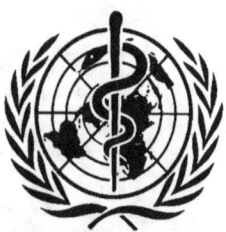

World Health Organization
Geneva 2000

WHO Library Cataloguing-in-Publication Data

WHO Consultation on Obesity (1999 : Geneva, Switzerland)
  Obesity : preventing and managing the global epidemic : report of a WHO consultation.

  (WHO technical report series ; 894)

  1.Obesity — epidemiology   2.Obesity — prevention and control   3.Cost of illness
  4.Nutrition policy   5.National health programs   I.Title   II.Series

  ISBN 92 4 120894 5   (NLM Classification : WD 710)
  ISSN 0512-3054

Typeset in Hong Kong
Printed in Singapore
99/12859 — Best-set/SNP — 6500
2004/15711 — Best-set/SNP — 500

Contents

WHO Consultation on Obesity

Geneva, 3–5 June 1997

Members*

Professor D-S. Akram, Department of Paediatrics, Dow Medical College, Civil Hospital, Karachi, Pakistan

Professor A.V. Astrup, Research Department of Human Nutrition, Royal Veterinary and Agricultural University, Copenhagen, Denmark

Professor T. Atinmo, Head, Department of Human Nutrition, College of Medicine, University of Ibadan, Ibadan, Nigeria

Dr J-L. Boissin, Director, Department of Endocrinology and Nutrition, Polynesian Institute of Research on Metabolic and Endocrine Disorders (IPRAME), Papeete, Tahiti, French Polynesia

Professor G.A. Bray, Executive Director, Pennington Biomedical Research Center, Louisiana State University, Baton Rouge, LA, USA

Dr K.K. Carroll, Director, Centre for Human Nutrition, Department of Biochemistry, University of Western Ontario, London, Ontario, Canada

Dr P. Chitson, Noncommunicable Diseases Office, Ministry of Health, Port Louis, Mauritius

Professor C. Chunming, Senior Advisor, Chinese Academy of Preventive Medicine, Beijing, China (*Vice-Chairman*)

Dr W.H. Dietz, Department of Pediatrics, Division of Gastroenterology and Nutrition, The Floating Hospital for Children, North-east Medical Centre, Boston, MA, USA

Dr J.O. Hill, Centre for Human Nutrition, University of Colorado, Denver, CO, USA (*Chairman*)

Professor E. Jéquier, Institute of Physiology, University of Lausanne, Lausanne, Switzerland

Dr C. Komodiki, Chief Health Officer, Ministry of Health, Nicosia, Cyprus

Professor Y. Matsuzawa, The Second Department of Internal Medicine, Osaka University School of Medicine, Osaka, Japan

Professor W.F. Mollentze, Department of Internal Medicine, University of the Orange Free State, Bloemfontein, South Africa

Dr K. Moosa, Head, Nutrition Unit, Ministry of Health, Manama, Bahrain

Dr M.I. Noor, Faculty of Allied Health Sciences, Kebangsaan Malaysia University, Kuala Lumpur, Malaysia

Dr K.S. Reddy, Department of Cardiology, Cardiothoracic Centre, All-India Institute of Medical Sciences, New Delhi, India

---

* Unable to attend: Professor M.J. Gibney, Department of Clinical Medicine, Trinity Centre for Health Sciences, St James's Hospital, Dublin, Ireland; Professor S. Rössner, Health Behaviour Research, Obesity Unit, Karolinska Hospital, Stockholm, Sweden; Dr F. Shaheen, Director, Nutrition Institute, Cairo, Egypt.

Dr J. Seidell, Department of Chronic Diseases and Environmental Epidemiology, National Institute of Public Health and Environment, Bilthoven, Netherlands (*Joint Rapporteur*)

Dr V. Tanphaichitr, Professor of Medicine and Deputy Dean for Academic Affairs, Faculty of Medicine, Ramathibodi Hospital, Mahidol University, Bangkok, Thailand

Dr R. Uauy, Director, Institute of Nutrition and Food Technology, University of Chile, Casilla, Santiago, Chile (*Joint Rapporteur*)

Professor P. Zimmet, Chief Executive Officer, International Diabetes Institute, Caulfield South, Victoria, Australia

Representatives of other organizations[†]

Administrative Committee on Coordination Subcommittee on Nutrition (ACC/SCN)

Dr S. Rabeneck, Technical Secretary, ACC/SCN, Geneva, Switzerland

Food and Agriculture Organization of the United Nations (FAO)

Dr G. Nantel, Senior Nutrition Officer, Food and Nutrition Division, FAO, Rome, Italy

WHO Collaborating Centres for Nutrition

Dr P. Deurenberg, Department of Human Nutrition and Epidemiology, Agricultural University, Wageningen, Netherlands

Dr M. Jarosz, Vice-Director, National Food and Nutrition Institute, Warsaw, Poland

Secretariat

Professor P. Björntorp, Department of Heart and Lung Diseases, University of Gothenburg Sahlgren's Hospital, Gothenburg, Sweden (*Temporary Adviser*)

Dr G.A. Clugston, Director, Programme of Nutrition, WHO, Geneva, Switzerland

Dr T. Gill, Scientific Secretary, International Obesity Task Force, Rowett Research Institute, Aberdeen, Scotland (*Temporary Adviser*)

Professor W.P.T. James, Chairman, International Obesity Task Force, Director, Rowett Research Institute, Aberdeen, Scotland (*Temporary Adviser*)

Dr N. Khaltaev, Responsible Officer, Division of Noncommunicable Diseases, WHO, Geneva, Switzerland (*Co-Secretary*)

Ms V. Lakin, Secretariat, International Obesity Task Force, Rowett Research Institute, Aberdeen, Scotland (*Temporary Adviser*)

Dr N.P. Napalkov, Assistant Director-General, WHO, Geneva, Switzerland

Mrs C. Nishida, Responsible Officer, Programme of Nutrition, WHO, Geneva, Switzerland (*Co-Secretary*)

Dr M. Peña, Regional Adviser in Food and Nutrition, WHO Regional Office for the Americas, WHO, Washington, DC, USA

[†] Invited but unable to send a representative: United Nations Children's Fund (UNICEF), New York, NY, USA; United Nations University (UNU), Tokyo, Japan.

Dr A. Robertson, Acting Regional Adviser, Nutrition Policy, Infant Feeding and Food Security Programme, WHO Regional Office for Europe, Copenhagen, Denmark

Dr M.S. Tsechkovski, Director, Division of Noncommunicable Diseases, WHO, Geneva, Switzerland

Dr T. Türmen, Executive Director, Family and Reproductive Health, WHO, Geneva, Switzerland

Abbreviations

The following abbreviations are used in this report:

AIHW	Australian Institute of Health and Welfare
ALCO	Anonymous Fighters Against Obesity (Argentina)
BMI	body mass index
BMR	basal metabolic rate
CHD	coronary heart disease
CHNS	China Health and Nutrition Survey
CHO	carbohydrate
CINDI	community interventions in noncommunicable diseases
CVD	cardiovascular disease
DALY	disability-adjusted life-year
DEXA	dual-energy X-ray absorptiometry
ENDEF	National Study of Family Expenditure (Brazil)
EPI	Expanded Programme on Immunization
EPOC	excess post-exercise oxygen consumption
FDA	Food and Drug Administration (USA)
HCG	human chorionic gonadotropin
HDL	high-density lipoprotein
HMR	health management resources
HPA	hypothalamic–pituitary axis
IGT	impaired glucose tolerance
INTERHEALTH	Integrated Programme for Community Health in Noncommunicable Diseases
INTERSALT	International Cooperative Study on the Relation of Blood Pressure to Electrolyte Excretion in Populations
IOTF	International Obesity Task Force
LDL	low-density lipoprotein
LDL-apoB	low-density lipoprotein apolipoprotein B
LMS	least mean square
LPL	lipoprotein lipase
MONICA	Monitoring of trends and determinants in cardiovascular diseases (WHO MONICA study)
NCD	noncommunicable disease
NCHS	National Center for Health Statistics (USA)
NEFA	non-esterified fatty acid
NHANES	National Health and Nutrition Examination Survey (USA)
NHES	National Health Examination Survey (USA)
NHMRC	National Health and Medical Research Council
NIDDM	non-insulin-dependent diabetes mellitus
NNS III	Third Nationwide Nutritional Survey in China (1992)
OA	Overeaters Anonymous
PAF	population-attributable fraction

PAL	physical activity level
PNSN	National Survey on Health and Nutrition (Brazil)
POP	Pound of Prevention
REDP	reduced-energy diet programme
RMR	resting metabolic rate
RR	relative risk
SBW	standard body weight
SHBG	sex hormone-binding globulin
SOS	Swedish Obese Subjects
SSRI	selective serotonin reuptake inhibitor
STD	sexually transmitted disease
TEF	thermic effect of food
TOPS	Taking Off Pounds Sensibly
VLCD	very-low-calorie diet
WHR	waist : hip circumference ratio or waist : hip ratio

1. Introduction

The WHO Consultation on Obesity met in Geneva from 3 to 5 June 1997. Dr F.S. Antezana, Deputy-Director General *ad interim*, opened the meeting on behalf of the Director-General. This consultation was the culmination of a two-year preparatory process, involving more than 100 experts worldwide, undertaken in close collaboration with the Rowett Research Institute (a WHO collaborating centre for nutrition) in Aberdeen, Scotland, and the International Obesity Task Force (IOTF) chaired by Professor Philip James, Director of the Rowett Research Institute.

The overall aim of the Consultation was to review current epidemiological information on obesity, and draw up recommendations for developing public health policies and programmes for improving the prevention and management of obesity. The specific objectives of the Consultation were:

— to review global prevalence and trends of obesity among children and adults, factors contributing to the problem of obesity, and associated consequences of obesity, such as chronic noncommunicable diseases;
— to examine health and economic consequences of obesity and their impact on development;
— to develop recommendations to assist countries in developing comprehensive public health policies and strategies for improving the prevention and management of obesity;
— to identify the issues requiring further research.

In order to achieve these objectives, six peer-reviewed background documents were prepared by experts in related fields. WHO takes pleasure in drawing attention to these contributions, in the absence of which many preparatory activities would not have been possible. The individuals and institutions that contributed are mentioned in the Acknowledgements section (page 251).

Throughout most of human history, weight gain and fat storage have been viewed as signs of health and prosperity. In times of hard labour and frequent food shortages, securing an adequate energy intake to meet requirements has been the major nutritional concern.

Today, however, as standards of living continue to rise, weight gain and obesity are posing a growing threat to health in countries all over the world. Obesity is a chronic disease, prevalent in both developed and developing countries, and affecting children as well as adults. Indeed, it is now so common that it is replacing the more traditional public health concerns, including undernutrition and infectious disease, as one of the most significant contributors to ill health. Furthermore, as obesity is a key risk factor in the natural history of other chronic and noncommunicable diseases (NCDs), it is only a matter of time before the same high mortality rates for such diseases will be seen in developing countries as those prevailing 30 years ago in industrialized countries with well established market economies.

Clinical evidence of obesity can be dated as far back as Graeco-Roman times, but little scientific progress was made towards understanding the condition until the 20th century. In the 19th century, the work of Lavoisier and others indicated that metabolism was similar to slow combustion, and that obese and lean humans obeyed the laws of thermodynamics. Also, the discovery that fat is stored in "cells", the basic units of biology, led to the idea that obesity could be caused by the presence of too many fat cells. Interestingly, the 19th century also saw the publication of the first diet book, entitled *Letter on corpulence addressed to the public*, by a Mr W. Banting.

In the early 20th century, analysis of life insurance data indicated that obesity was associated with an increased death rate. A familial basis for obesity was suggested in the 1920s, and Cushing disease and hypothalamic obesity were described. Later, the introduction of thyroid hormone, dinitrophenol and amfetamine as pharmacological treatments for obesity opened the door to the use of drugs, and genetics improved the understanding of several specific forms of obesity resulting from genetic defects.

Considerable advances have been made in diet, exercise and behavioural approaches to treatment for obesity since their advent in the first half of the 20th century, and new drugs with ever-better profiles of pharmacological activity continue to be introduced on a regular basis. Gastric surgery has had the most effective long-term success in treating the severely obese. Despite this progress, however, obesity prevalence continues to increase sharply, and the challenge to public health workers and scientists has never been greater.

This report provides an assessment of current data on the prevalence of obesity, its health consequences and its economic costs. Strategies for implementing a systematic approach to the prevention and management of obesity in different health service systems are described, and recommendations by leading international obesity experts are also given. It is hoped that these recommendations will be used in the development of new policies to address the escalating public health problem of obesity.

1.1 Structure of the report

The report is divided into five parts, the first four of which deal with different aspects of the global epidemic of obesity. The final part outlines the conclusions and recommendations of the WHO Consultation on Obesity.

Part I examines the definition and classification of obesity, and sets out the most recent data on the global prevalence and secular trends in all regions of the world. Defining and identifying the extent of the problem of obesity is a critical first step in a coherent approach to its prevention and management.

Part II covers the true costs of obesity in terms of physical and mental ill health, and the human and financial resources diverted to deal with the problem. The amount of suffering that obesity causes, and the money spent by health agencies in dealing with it, are enormous and reinforce the need for urgent action.

Part III examines what is known about this complex, multifactorial disease and identifies the major factors implicated in its development. Most of the information about risk factors for weight gain and obesity comes from studies in developed countries because developing countries have only recently seen a rise in chronic diseases and therefore have little experience in carrying out research in this area. Examination of the factors involved in weight gain and obesity in developed countries, however, is of worldwide relevance in predicting the future impact in countries in the early stages of frequently dramatic socio-economic change and provides a unique opportunity for taking preventive action. It is also important that these factors should be taken into account in any coordinated strategy designed to tackle the problem of obesity.

Part IV takes account of the matters considered in the preceding three parts and presents the foundations of a comprehensive strategy for the prevention and management of obesity through health care services and public health policy. Policy-makers, health professionals and the community at large need to join forces in tackling this major global public health problem.

Part V outlines the final conclusions and recommendations of the WHO Consultation on Obesity. Priority areas for further research are identified, and recommendations on strategies and actions for the effective prevention and management of the global epidemic of obesity are made.

1.2 Themes of the report

Obesity is a complex and incompletely understood disease. This report highlights key issues central to the development of a coherent strategy for the effective prevention and management of obesity on a worldwide basis. A number of important themes have dictated the content and style of the report, including the following:

- Obesity is a serious disease, but its development is not inevitable. It is largely preventable through lifestyle changes.

- The health risks of excessive body fat are associated with a relatively small increase in body weight, not only with marked obesity. Effective management of obesity cannot be separated from prevention.

- Obesity is not just an individual problem. It is a population problem and should be tackled as such. Effective prevention and management of obesity will require an integrated approach, involving actions in all sectors of society.

- Obesity is a chronic disease that requires long-term strategies for its effective prevention and management.

- Obesity affects all age groups. The effective prevention of adult obesity will require the prevention and management of childhood obesity.

- Obesity is a global problem. Prevention and management strategies applicable to all regions of the world should be developed.

- Obesity can be seen as just one of a defined cluster of noncommunicable diseases (NCDs) now observed in both developed and developing countries. The global epidemic of obesity is a reflection of the massive social, economic and cultural problems currently facing developing and newly industrialized countries, as well as the ethnic minorities and the disadvantaged in developed countries.

- Examination of the factors involved in weight gain and obesity in developed countries is crucial for predictions about the future impact in countries in the early stages of frequently dramatic socioeconomic change and provides a unique opportunity for taking preventive action.

- In countries with developing economies, the problem of obesity is emerging at a time when undernutrition remains a significant problem. Strategies that take account of both these important nutritional problems will need to be developed, particularly when dealing with children whose growth may be stunted.

PART I

The problem of overweight and obesity

2. Defining the problem

2.1 Introduction

Obesity is often defined simply as a condition of abnormal or excessive fat accumulation in adipose tissue, to the extent that health may be impaired (*1*). The underlying disease is the undesirable positive energy balance and weight gain. However, obese individuals differ not only in the amount of excess fat that they store, but also in the regional distribution of that fat within the body. The distribution of fat induced by weight gain affects the risks associated with obesity, and the kinds of disease that result. Indeed, excess abdominal fat is as great a risk factor for disease as is excess body fat *per se*. It is useful, therefore, to be able to distinguish between those at increased risk as a result of "abdominal fat distribution", or "android obesity" as it is often known, from those with the less serious "gynoid" fat distribution, in which fat is more evenly and peripherally distributed around the body.

Classifying obesity during childhood or adolescence is further complicated by the fact that height is still increasing and body composition is continually changing. Furthermore, there are substantial international differences in the age of onset of puberty and in the differential interindividual rates of fat accumulation.

This section outlines the most appropriate methods for: (a) classifying overweight and obesity in adults; and (b) identifying abdominal fat distribution. It also briefly discusses the use of additional tools for use in the more detailed characterization of obese individuals. The final section outlines the current lack of consistency and agreement between studies in the classification of obesity in childhood and adolescence, and highlights the need for a globally standardized classification system.

The key issues covered include the following:

- Obesity can be defined simply as the disease in which excess body fat has accumulated to such an extent that health may be adversely affected. However, the amount of excess fat, its distribution within the body, and the associated health consequences vary considerably between obese individuals.

- The graded classification of overweight and obesity: (a) permits meaningful comparisons of weight status within and between populations; (b) makes it possible to identify individuals and groups at increased risk of morbidity and mortality; (c) enables priorities to be identified for intervention at individual and community levels; and (d) provides a firm basis for the evaluation of interventions.

- Body mass index (BMI) (see section 2.3) provides the most useful, albeit crude, population-level measure of obesity. It can be used to estimate the prevalence of obesity within a population and the risks associated with it. However, BMI does not account for the wide variation in body fat distribution, and may not correspond to the same degree of fatness or associated health risk in different individuals and populations.

- Obese individuals with excess fat in the intra-abdominal depots are at particular risk of the adverse health consequences of obesity. Therefore, measurement of waist circumference provides a simple and practical method of identifying overweight patients at increased risk of obesity-associated illness due to abdominal fat distribution.

- Ethnic populations differ in the level of risk associated with a particular waist circumference, and a globally applicable grading system of waist circumference has not yet been developed.

- Additional tools available for the more detailed characterization of the obese state include methods of measuring body composition (e.g. underwater weighing), determining the anatomical distribution of body fat (e.g. magnetic resonance imaging), and measuring energy intake (e.g. prospective dietary record) and energy expenditure (e.g. doubly labelled water). However, the cost of such techniques and the practical difficulties involved in applying them limit their usefulness to research.

- As previously mentioned, the classification of the weight status of children and adolescents is complicated by the fact that height and body composition are continually changing, and that such changes often occur at different rates and times in different populations, making simple universal indices of adiposity of little value. To date, there has not been the same level of agreement on the classification of obesity for children and adolescents as there is for adults.

2.2 Why classify overweight and obesity?

The graded classification of overweight and obesity is valuable for a number of reasons. In particular, it allows:

- meaningful comparisons of weight status within and between populations;
- the identification of individuals and groups at increased risk of morbidity and mortality;
- the identification of priorities for intervention at individual and community levels;
- a firm basis for evaluating interventions.

2.3 Body mass index

BMI is a simple index of weight-for-height that is commonly used to classify underweight, overweight and obesity in adults. It is defined as the weight in kilograms divided by the square of the height in metres (kg/m^2).

For example, an adult who weighs 70 kg and whose height is 1.75 m will have a BMI of 22.9:

$$BMI = 70(kg)/1.75^2 (m^2) = 22.9$$

The classification of overweight and obesity, according to BMI, is shown in Table 2.1. Obesity is classified as a BMI $\geq$30.0. The classification shown in Table 2.1 is in agreement with that recommended by WHO (2), but includes an additional subdivision at BMI 35.0–39.9 in recognition of the fact that management options for dealing with obesity differ above a BMI of 35. The WHO classification is based primarily on the association between BMI and mortality (see section 4.6).

2.3.1 *Use of other cut-off points in the classification of obesity*

A BMI of 30 or more is now widely accepted as denoting obesity. In some studies, however, other BMI cut-off points both above and below 30 have been used (3). Differences in cut-off points have a major impact on estimates of the prevalence of obesity. For meaningful comparisons between or within populations it is therefore advisable to use the single BMI cut-off points proposed in Table 2.1.

2.3.2 *Variation in the relationship between BMI and body fatness*

Although it can generally be assumed that individuals with a BMI of 30 or above have an excess fat mass in their body, BMI does not distinguish between weight associated with muscle and weight associated with fat. As a result, the relationship between BMI and body fat content varies according to body build and proportion, and it has been shown repeatedly that a given BMI may not correspond to the same degree of fatness across populations. Polynesians, for example, tend to have a lower fat percentage than Caucasian Australians at an identical BMI (4). In addition, the percentage of body fat mass increases with age up to 60–65 years in both sexes (5, 6), and is higher in women than in men of equivalent BMI (7). In cross-sectional comparisons, therefore, BMI values should be interpreted with caution if estimates of body fat are required.

Differences in body proportions and in the relationship between BMI and body fat content can affect the BMI range considered to be healthy. Calculations based on the ratio of sitting height to standing

Table 2.1
Classification of adults according to BMI[a]

Classification	BMI	Risk of comorbidities
Underweight	<18.50	Low (but risk of other clinical problems increased)
Normal range	18.50–24.99	Average
Overweight:	≥25.00	
Preobese	25.00–29.99	Increased
Obese class I	30.00–34.99	Moderate
Obese class II	35.00–39.99	Severe
Obese class III	≥40.00	Very severe

[a] These BMI values are age-independent and the same for both sexes. However, BMI may not correspond to the same degree of fatness in different populations due, in part, to differences in body proportions (see section 2.3.2). The table shows a simplistic relationship between BMI and the risk of comorbidity, which can be affected by a range of factors, including the nature of the diet, ethnic group and activity level. The risks associated with increasing BMI are continuous and graded and begin at a BMI above 25. The interpretation of BMI gradings in relation to risk may differ for different populations. Both BMI and a measure of fat distribution (waist circumference or waist : hip ratio (WHR)) are important in calculating the risk of obesity comorbidities.

height that allow BMI to be corrected to take account of unusual leg lengths are now available. Thus, very tall and lean Australian Aboriginals tend to have a deceptively low BMI; a healthy BMI range for this population appears to be between 17 and 22, metabolic complications developing rapidly as BMI increases above 22. Recalculating Aboriginal data to allow for their unusual body proportions increases both the mean BMI and the BMI distribution, so that the percentage with a BMI >25 increases from 8% to 15% (8).

2.3.3 *Use of BMI to classify obesity*

BMI can be considered to provide the most useful, albeit crude, population-level measure of obesity. The robust nature of the measurements and the widespread routine inclusion of weights and heights in clinical and population health surveys mean that a more selective measure of adiposity, such as skinfold thickness measurements, provides additional rather than primary information. BMI can be used to estimate the prevalence of obesity within a population and the risks associated with it, but does not, however, account for the wide variation in the nature of obesity between different individuals and populations.

2.4 **Waist circumference and waist:hip ratio**

Abdominal fat mass can vary dramatically within a narrow range of total body fat or BMI. Indeed, for any accumulation of total body fat, men have on average twice the amount of abdominal fat than is generally found in premenopausal women (9). Other methods in addition to the measurement of BMI would therefore be valuable in identifying individuals at increased risk from obesity-related illness due to abdominal fat accumulation.

Over the past 10 years or so, it has become accepted that a high WHR (WHR >1.0 in men and >0.85 in women) indicates abdominal fat accumulation (10). However, recent evidence suggests that waist circumference alone — measured at the midpoint between the lower border of the rib cage and the iliac crest — may provide a more practical correlate of abdominal fat distribution and associated ill health (11–13).

Waist circumference is a convenient and simple measurement that is unrelated to height (10), correlates closely with BMI and WHR (13) and is an approximate index of intra-abdominal fat mass (14–16) and total body fat (17). Furthermore, changes in waist circumference reflect changes in risk factors for cardiovascular disease (CVD) (18) and other forms of chronic disease, even though the risks seem to vary in different populations.

Some experts consider that the hip measurement provides additional valuable information related to gluteofemoral muscle mass and bone structure (19). The WHR may therefore remain a useful research tool, but individuals can be identified as being at increased risk of obesity-related illness by using waist circumference alone as an initial screening tool.

Populations differ in the level of risk associated with a particular waist circumference, so that globally applicable cut-off points cannot be developed. For instance, abdominal fatness has been shown to be less strongly associated with risk factors for CVD and non-insulin-dependent diabetes mellitus (NIDDM) in black women than in white women (20). Also, people of South Asian (Bangladeshi, Indian and Pakistani) descent living in urban societies have a higher prevalence of many of the complications of obesity than other ethnic groups (21). These complications are associated with abdominal fat distribution that is markedly higher for a given level of BMI than in Europeans. Finally, although women have almost the same absolute risk of coronary heart disease (CHD) as men at the same WHR (22, 23), they show increases in relative risk of CHD at lower waist circumferences than men. Thus, there is a need to develop sex-specific waist circumference cut-off points appropriate for different populations.

Table 2.2
Sex-specific waist circumference and risk of metabolic complications associated with obesity in Caucasians[a]

Risk of metabolic complications	Waist circumference (cm)	
	Men	Women
Increased	≥94	≥80
Substantially increased	≥102	≥88

[a] This table is an example only. The identification of risk using waist circumference is population-specific and will depend on levels of obesity and other risk factors for CVD and NIDDM. This issue is currently under investigation.

The sex-specific waist circumferences given in Table 2.2 denote enhanced relative risk for a random sample from the Netherlands of 2183 men and 2698 women aged 20–59 years (*23*).

2.5 Additional tools for the assessment of obesity

In addition to the anthropometric assessment methods previously outlined, there are various other tools that are useful for measuring body fat in certain clinical situations and in obesity research. These tools are particularly useful when trying to identify the genetic and environmental determinants of obesity and their interactions, as they enable the variable and complex nature of obesity to be split up into separate components. Thus, obese individuals can be characterized by measuring body composition, anatomical distribution of fat, energy intake, and insulin resistance, among others.

A list of those characteristics of obesity considered suitable for measuring in genetic studies has recently been agreed (*24*) and is summarized in Table 2.3. Measures in a given category are not necessarily of equal validity.

2.6 Classifying obesity in childhood

To date, there has not been the same level of agreement over the classification of overweight and obesity in children and adolescents as in adults. There has been confusion both in terms of a globally applicable reference population and of the selection of appropriate cut-off points for designating a child as obese.

2.6.1 *Use of growth charts*

Many countries have produced reference charts for growth based on weight-for-age and height-for-age. However, these measures are a reflection only of the child's size (height and girth) and provide no indication of relative fatness. The close correlation between height

Table 2.3
Currently recommended characteristics for measurement in genetic studies

Characteristic of obesity measured	Examples of measurement tools
Body composition	BMI; waist circumference; underwater weighing; dual-energy X-ray absorptiometry (DEXA); isotope dilution; bioelectrical impedance; skinfold thickness
Anatomical distribution of fat	Waist circumference; WHR; computer tomography; ultrasound; magnetic resonance imaging
Partitioning of nutrient storage	$[^{13}C]$ palmitic acid; extended overfeeding challenge
Energy intake	"Total" by prospective dietary record or recall; "macronutrient composition" by prospective dietary record or recall or by dietary questionnaire
Energy expenditure	"Total" by double-labelled water; "resting" by indirect calorimetry; physical activity level (PAL) by questionnaire, motion detector, heart-rate monitor, etc.

and weight during childhood means that an index of weight adjusted for height can provide a simple measure of fatness.

2.6.2 *International childhood reference population*

The most widely used growth reference, which WHO has recommended for international use since the late 1970s (*25, 26*), was developed by the US National Center for Health Statistics (NCHS). However, a WHO Expert Committee (*2*) has drawn attention to a number of serious technical and biological problems with this growth reference. WHO is therefore currently undertaking the development of a new growth reference for infants and children from birth to 5 years. This will be based on a sample of infants and children from different parts of the world whose caregivers follow internationally recognized health recommendations. A similar reference will also be required for older children and adolescents.

2.6.3 *BMI-for-age reference curves*

Adult BMI increases very slowly with age, so age-independent cut-off points can be used to grade fatness. In children, however, BMI changes substantially with age, rising steeply in infancy, falling during the preschool years, and then rising again during adolescence and early adulthood. For this reason, child BMI needs to be assessed using age-related reference curves.

Such curves have been produced for a number of countries (6, 27–29). However, many are imperfect either because the data are old or because the age range is restricted. More recent BMI-for-age charts have been developed for British, Italian and Swedish children (30–32) using the least mean square (LMS) method of Cole (33), which adjusts BMI distribution for skewness and allows BMI in individual subjects to be expressed as an exact centile or standard deviation score. The use of BMI-for-age is currently being explored, in parallel with other potential techniques, by an expert working group in order to determine the best method of classifying overweight and obesity in childhood. A common standard should allow the comparative evaluation of childhood obesity internationally.

References

1. Garrow JS. *Obesity and related diseases*. London, Churchill Livingstone, 1988:1–16.

2. *Physical status: the use and interpretation of anthropometry. Report of a WHO Expert Committee*. Geneva, World Health Organization, 1995 (Technical Report Series, No. 854):329.

3. Kuczmarski RJ et al. Increasing prevalence of overweight among US adults. The National Health and Nutrition Examination Surveys, 1960 to 1991. *Journal of the American Medical Association*, 1994, **272**:205–211.

4. Swinburn BA et al. Body composition differences between Polynesians and Caucasians assessed by bioelectrical impedance. *International Journal of Obesity and Related Metabolic Disorders*, 1996, **20**:889–894.

5. Forbes GB, Reina JC. Adult lean body mass decline with age: some longitudinal observations. *Metabolism: Clinical and Experimental*, 1970, **19**:653–663.

6. Rolland-Cachera MF et al. Body mass index variations — centiles from birth to 87 years. *European Journal of Clinical Nutrition*, 1991, **45**:13–21.

7. Ross R et al. Sex differences in lean and adipose tissue distribution by magnetic resonance imaging: anthropometric relationships. *American Journal of Clinical Nutrition*, 1994, **59**:1277–1285.

8. Norgan NG, Jones PRM. The effect of standardising the body mass index for relative sitting height. *International Journal of Obesity and Related Metabolic Disorders*, 1995, **19**:206–208.

9. Lemieux S et al. Sex differences in the relation of visceral adipose tissue accumulation to total body fatness. *American Journal of Clinical Nutrition*, 1993, **58**:463–467.

10. Han TS et al. The influences of height and age on waist circumferences as an index of adiposity in adults. *International Journal of Obesity and Related Metabolic Disorders*, 1997, **21**:83–89.

11. **James WPT.** The epidemiology of obesity. In: Chadwick DJ, Cardew GC, eds. *The origins and consequences of obesity.* Chichester, Wiley, 1996:1–16 (Ciba Foundation Symposium 201).

12. **Seidell JC.** Are abdominal diameters abominable indicators? In: Angel A, Bouchard C, eds. *Progress in Obesity Research: 7.* London, Libbey, 1995:305–308.

13. **Lean MEJ, Han TS, Morrison CE.** Waist circumference as a measure for indicating need for weight management. *British Medical Journal,* 1995, **311**:158–161.

14. **Han TS et al.** Waist circumference relates to intra-abdominal fat mass better than waist:hip ratio in women. *Proceedings of the Nutrition Society,* 1995, **54**:152A.

15. **Pouliot MC et al.** Waist circumference and abdominal sagittal diameter: best simple anthropometric indexes of abdominal visceral adipose tissue accumulation and related cardiovascular risk in men and women. *American Journal of Cardiology,* 1994, **73**:460–468.

16. **Ross R et al.** Quantification of adipose tissue by MRI: relationship with anthropometric variables. *Journal of Applied Physiology,* 1992, **72**:787–795.

17. **Lean MEJ, Han TS, Deurenberg P.** Predicting body composition by densitometry from simple anthropometric measurements. *American Journal of Clinical Nutrition,* 1996, **63**:4–14.

18. **Han TS et al.** Waist circumference reduction and cardiovascular benefits during weight loss in women. *International Journal of Obesity and Related Metabolic Disorders,* 1997, **21**:127–134.

19. **Björntorp P.** Etiology of the metabolic syndrome. In: Bray GA, Bouchard C, James WPT, eds. *Handbook of obesity.* New York, Marcel Dekker, 1998:573–600.

20. **Dowling HJ, Pi-Sunyer FX.** Race-dependent health risks of upper body obesity. *Diabetes,* 1993, **42**:537–543.

21. **McKeigue PM.** Metabolic consequences of obesity and body fat pattern: lessons from migrant studies. In: Chadwick DJ, Cardew GC, eds. *The origins and consequences of obesity.* Chichester, Wiley, 1996:54–67 (Ciba Foundation Symposium 201).

22. **Larsson B et al.** Is abdominal body fat distribution a major explanation for the sex difference in the incidence of myocardial infarction? The study of men born in 1913 and the study of women, Göteborg, Sweden. *American Journal of Epidemiology,* 1992, **135**:266–273.

23. **Han TS et al.** Waist circumference action levels in the identification of cardiovascular risk factors: prevalence study in a random sample. *British Medical Journal,* 1995, **311**:1401–1405.

24. **Warden CH.** Group report: How can we best apply the tools of genetics to study body weight regulation? In: Bouchard C, Bray GA, eds. *Regulation of body weight: biological and behavioural mechanisms.* Chichester, Wiley, 1996:285–305.

25. *Measuring change in nutritional status.* Geneva, World Health Organization, 1983.

26. **WHO Working Group.** Use and interpretation of anthropometric indicators of nutritional status. *Bulletin of the World Health Organization*, 1986, **64**:929–941.

27. **Must A, Dallal GE, Dietz WH.** Reference data for obesity: 85th and 95th percentiles of body mass index and triceps skinfold thickness. *American Journal of Clinical Nutrition*, 1991, **53**:839–846.

28. **Hammer LD et al.** Standardized percentile curves of body mass index for children and adolescents. *American Journal of Diseases of Children*, 1991, **145**:259–263.

29. **Bláha P et al.** V. celostátní antropologický výzkum detí a mládeze v roce 1991 (České zeme) — vybrané antropometrické charakteristiky. [The 5th nationwide anthropological study of children and adolescents held in 1991 (Czech Republic) — selected anthropometric characteristics.] *Československa Pediatrie*, 1993, **48**(10):621–630.

30. **Cole TJ, Freeman JV, Preece MA.** Body mass index reference curves for the UK, 1990. *Archives of Diseases of Children*, 1995, **73**:25–29.

31. **Luciano A, Bressan F, Zoppi G.** Body mass index reference curves for children aged 3–19 years from Verona, Italy. *European Journal of Clinical Nutrition*, 1997, **51**:6–10.

32. **Lindgren G et al.** Swedish population reference standards for height, weight and body mass index attained at 6 to 16 years (girls) or 19 years (boys). *Acta Paediatrica*, 1995, **84**(9):1019–1028.

33. **Cole TJ.** The LMS method for constructing normalised growth standards. *European Journal of Clinical Nutrition*, 1990, **44**:45–60.

3. Global prevalence and secular trends in obesity

3.1 Introduction

Evidence is now emerging to suggest that the prevalence of over-weight and obesity is increasing worldwide at an alarming rate. Both developed and developing countries are affected. Moreover, as the problem appears to be increasing rapidly in children as well as in adults, the true health consequences may only become fully apparent in the future.

The value of estimating the prevalence of, and secular trends in, overweight and obesity cannot be overemphasized. Knowledge of the level and changing distribution of overweight and obesity can be used to:

— identify populations at particular risk of obesity and its associated health and economic consequences;
— help policy-makers and public health planners in the mobilization and reallocation of resources for the control of disease;
— provide baseline data for monitoring the effectiveness of national programmes for the control of obesity.

This section provides a global overview of secular trends in obesity among adults. It begins with a note of caution on comparisons be-tween different studies, and then outlines the results of the compre-hensive WHO MONICA (MONItoring of trends and determinants in CArdiovascular diseases) study. The bulk of the section, however, is a review of secular trends over the past 10–20 years and the most recent prevalence data available within each of the six WHO regions — Africa, the Americas, South-East Asia, Europe, the Eastern Medi-terranean and the Western Pacific.

Despite the limited availability of nationally representative data (par-ticularly secular trend data), the following conclusions can be drawn:

• Obesity prevalence is increasing worldwide at an alarming rate in both developed and developing countries.

• In many developing countries, obesity coexists with undernutrition (BMI <18.5). It is still relatively uncommon in African and Asian countries, but is more prevalent in urban than in rural populations. In economically advanced regions, prevalence rates may be as high as in industrialized countries.

• Women generally have higher rates of obesity than men, although men may have higher rates of overweight.

• The current lack of consistency and agreement between different studies in the classification of obesity in children and adolescents makes it difficult to give an overview of the global prevalence of obesity in younger age groups. Nevertheless, irrespective of the classification system used, studies of obesity during childhood and adolescence have generally reported that its prevalence has increased.

3.2 A note of caution

Several factors can make comparisons of data between different cross-sectional studies problematic, namely:

- *Classification of obesity*: in a number of studies, the recommended WHO international classification of obesity, i.e. BMI ≥30, has not been used.

- *Age group*: the age group chosen affects the proportion of obese individuals identified.

- *Age standardization*: in many studies, the age structure of the population has not been standardized according to a reference such as the new standard world population data (*1*).

- *Time period/year of data collection*: there is a need for the continuous monitoring of programmes so that current data are always available.

- *Measured versus self-reported weight and height*: self-reported weight and height are notoriously unreliable, especially in the obese.

Many studies have been excluded from this review because of problems caused by the factors listed above, or because they were conducted several years ago without any follow-up and are therefore of limited value. The prevalence data cited in this section are those most recently available and illustrate the global nature of the prevalence of obesity; they have generally been derived from representative national surveys. However, due to the limited availability of longitudinal data, secular trends have often been illustrated with data from representative samples.

In all the tables in this section, obesity is classified as BMI ≥ 30 unless otherwise stated.

3.3 The WHO MONICA project

The most comprehensive data on the prevalence of obesity worldwide are those of the WHO MONICA project (*2*). Although the populations are not necessarily representative of the countries in which they are located, the 48 populations shown in Figs 3.1 and 3.2 can be

Figure 3.1

BMI distribution: age-standardized proportions of selected categories in MONICA populations, age group 35–64 years (men)

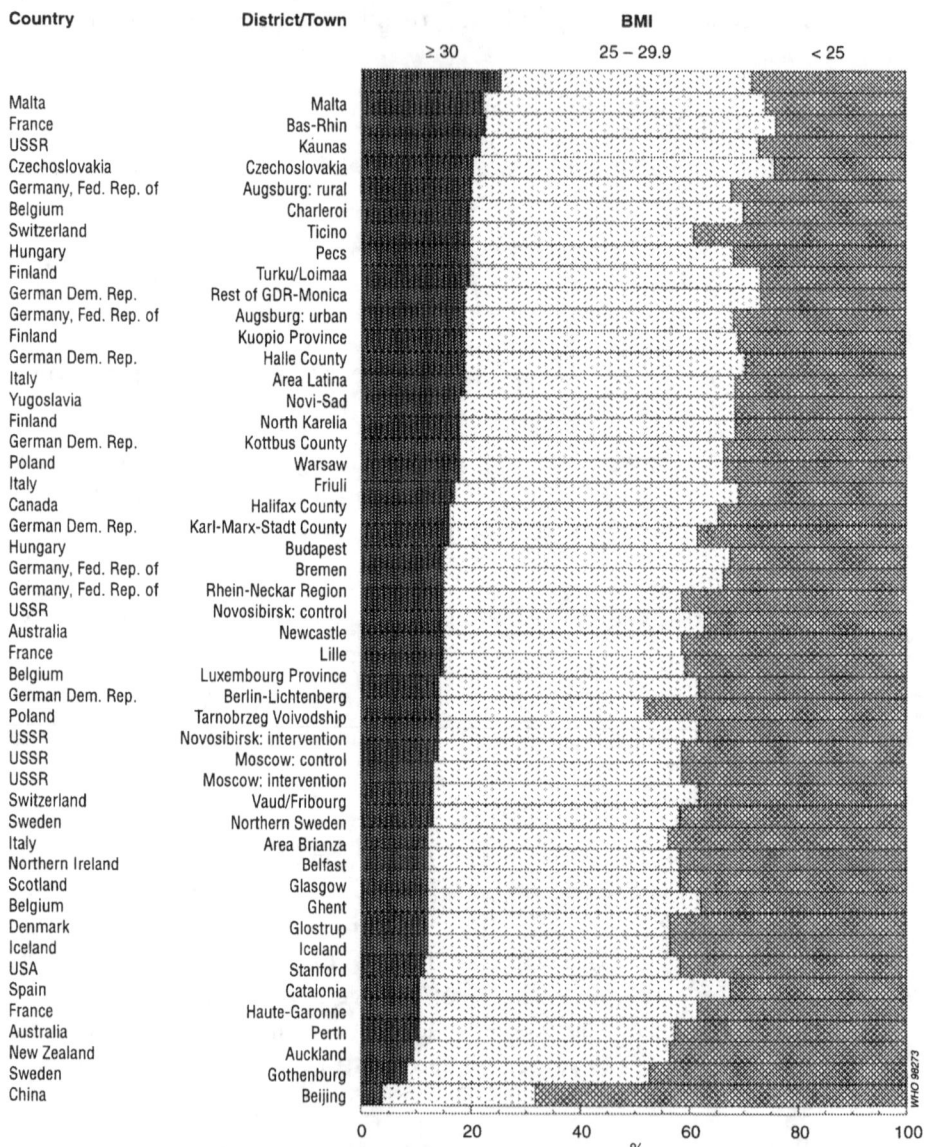

Country	District/Town
Malta	Malta
France	Bas-Rhin
USSR	Kaunas
Czechoslovakia	Czechoslovakia
Germany, Fed. Rep. of	Augsburg: rural
Belgium	Charleroi
Switzerland	Ticino
Hungary	Pecs
Finland	Turku/Loimaa
German Dem. Rep.	Rest of GDR-Monica
Germany, Fed. Rep. of	Augsburg: urban
Finland	Kuopio Province
German Dem. Rep.	Halle County
Italy	Area Latina
Yugoslavia	Novi-Sad
Finland	North Karelia
German Dem. Rep.	Kottbus County
Poland	Warsaw
Italy	Friuli
Canada	Halifax County
German Dem. Rep.	Karl-Marx-Stadt County
Hungary	Budapest
Germany, Fed. Rep. of	Bremen
Germany, Fed. Rep. of	Rhein-Neckar Region
USSR	Novosibirsk: control
Australia	Newcastle
France	Lille
Belgium	Luxembourg Province
German Dem. Rep.	Berlin-Lichtenberg
Poland	Tarnobrzeg Voivodship
USSR	Novosibirsk: intervention
USSR	Moscow: control
USSR	Moscow: intervention
Switzerland	Vaud/Fribourg
Sweden	Northern Sweden
Italy	Area Brianza
Northern Ireland	Belfast
Scotland	Glasgow
Belgium	Ghent
Denmark	Glostrup
Iceland	Iceland
USA	Stanford
Spain	Catalonia
France	Haute-Garonne
Australia	Perth
New Zealand	Auckland
Sweden	Gothenburg
China	Beijing

BMI: ≥ 30 | 25 – 29.9 | < 25

WHO 98273

Note 1. The proportions of men classified as obese, overweight and normal weight in 48 populations (mainly European) taking part in the WHO MONICA study are shown. Although these populations are not necessarily representative of the countries in which they are located, they can be compared because the data were collected in the same time period, are age-standardized, and are based on heights and weights measured in accordance with identical protocols. The WHO MONICA study has generated one of the most comprehensive data sets on the prevalence of obesity worldwide. The data were collected over the period 1983–1986 (*3*).

Note 2. Names of countries are those that were valid at the time of data collection.

Figure 3.2

BMI distribution: age-standardized proportions of selected categories in MONICA populations, age group 35–64 years (women)

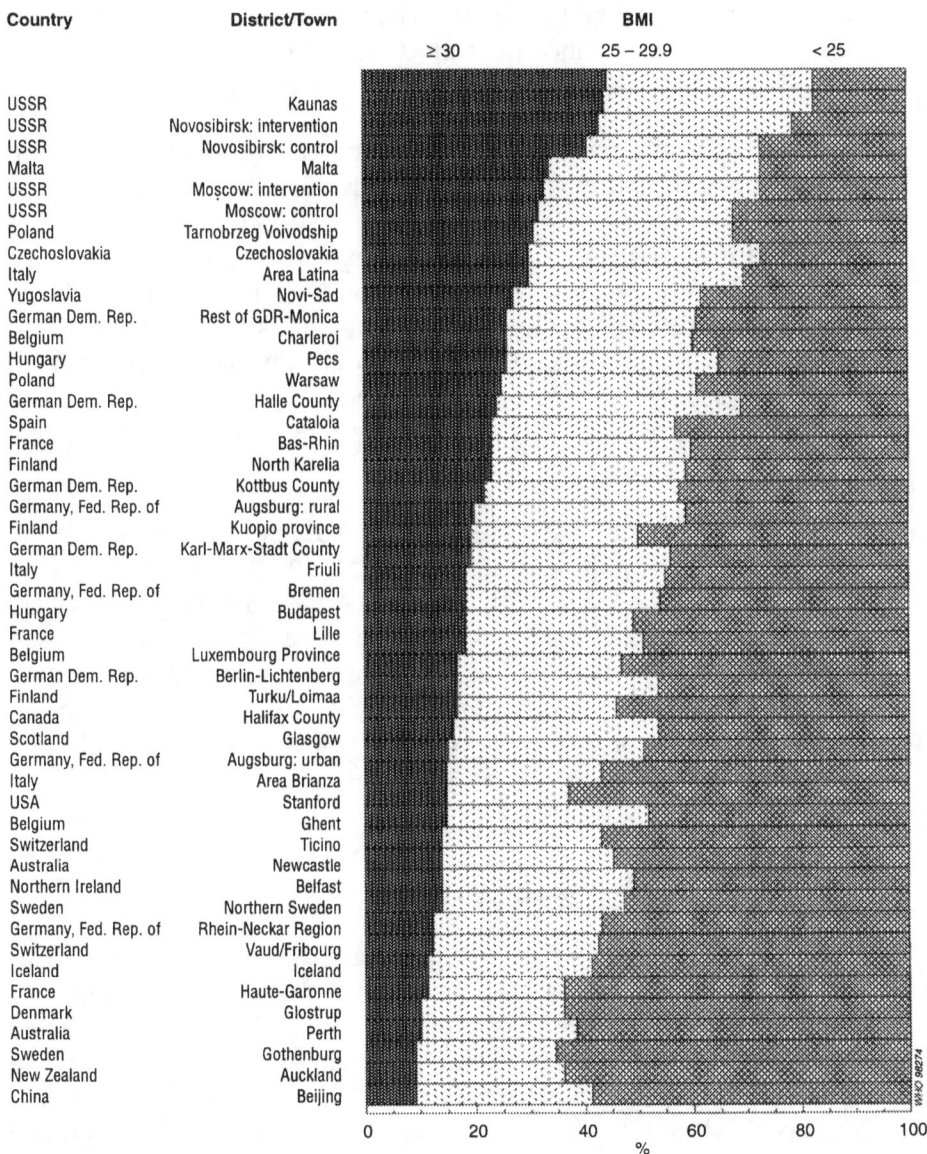

Country	District/Town	BMI
		≥ 30 25 – 29.9 < 25
USSR	Kaunas	
USSR	Novosibirsk: intervention	
USSR	Novosibirsk: control	
Malta	Malta	
USSR	Moscow: intervention	
USSR	Moscow: control	
Poland	Tarnobrzeg Voivodship	
Czechoslovakia	Czechoslovakia	
Italy	Area Latina	
Yugoslavia	Novi-Sad	
German Dem. Rep.	Rest of GDR-Monica	
Belgium	Charleroi	
Hungary	Pecs	
Poland	Warsaw	
German Dem. Rep.	Halle County	
Spain	Cataloia	
France	Bas-Rhin	
Finland	North Karelia	
German Dem. Rep.	Kottbus County	
Germany, Fed. Rep. of	Augsburg: rural	
Finland	Kuopio province	
German Dem. Rep.	Karl-Marx-Stadt County	
Italy	Friuli	
Germany, Fed. Rep. of	Bremen	
Hungary	Budapest	
France	Lille	
Belgium	Luxembourg Province	
German Dem. Rep.	Berlin-Lichtenberg	
Finland	Turku/Loimaa	
Canada	Halifax County	
Scotland	Glasgow	
Germany, Fed. Rep. of	Augsburg: urban	
Italy	Area Brianza	
USA	Stanford	
Belgium	Ghent	
Switzerland	Ticino	
Australia	Newcastle	
Northern Ireland	Belfast	
Sweden	Northern Sweden	
Germany, Fed. Rep. of	Rhein-Neckar Region	
Switzerland	Vaud/Fribourg	
Iceland	Iceland	
France	Haute-Garonne	
Denmark	Glostrup	
Australia	Perth	
Sweden	Gothenburg	
New Zealand	Auckland	
China	Beijing	

0   20   40   60   80   100
%

WHO 98274

Note 1. The proportions of women classified as obese, overweight and normal weight in 48 populations (mainly European) taking part in the WHO MONICA study are shown. Although these populations are not necessarily representative of the countries in which they are located, they can be compared because the data were collected in the same time period, are age-standardized, and are based on heights and weights measured in accordance with identical protocols. The WHO MONICA study has generated one of the most comprehensive data sets on the prevalence of obesity worldwide. The data were collected over the period 1983–1986 (*3*).

Note 2. Names of countries are those that were valid at the time of data collection.

compared because the data were collected in the same time period, are age-standardized, and are based on weights and heights measured in accordance with identical protocols. The data presented were collected in the first round between 1983 and 1986, and more recent data have been published since the time of the WHO Consultation.[1] The majority of the data are for European populations.

Figs 3.1 and 3.2 show the BMI distributions in 48 MONICA populations for men and women, respectively (3). Although this report focuses on data relating to obesity, i.e. BMI ≥30, it is important to note that a BMI between 25 and 29.9 is responsible for the major part of the impact of overweight on certain obesity comorbidities; it has been estimated, for example, that about 64% of male and 77% of female cases of NIDDM would theoretically be prevented if no one had a BMI ≥25. These figures may be compared with those for a BMI cut-off point of less than 30, namely 44% and 33%, respectively (4, 5).

Figs 3.1 and 3.2 show that, in all but one male population, and in the majority of female populations, between 50% and 75% of adults aged 35–64 years were either overweight or obese during the period 1983–1986. In a few populations, this figure was over 75%. Thus, between 1983 and 1986, the majority of adults in these populations were at increased risk of illness due to overweight or obesity. Based on the evidence that the prevalence of obesity is increasing worldwide, the situation is now likely to be even worse.

3.4 African Region

3.4.1 Secular trends in obesity

Many countries in the African Region have necessarily focused principally on undernutrition and food security. As a result, trends in obesity have been documented in only a few African countries or populations. However, one recent study in Mauritius has shown the same trend as that seen in the other five WHO regions — a dramatic increase in obesity prevalence over a five-year period in both men and women aged 25–74 years. The proportion of obese men increased from 3.4% in 1987 to 5.3% in 1992, while the proportion of obese women increased from 10.4% to 15.2% in the same period. This increase was seen in all age groups and ethnic groups (6, 7). Although

---

[1] Tunstall-Pedoe H et al. Contribution of trends in survival and coronary-event rates to changes in coronary heart disease mortality: 10 year results from 37 WHO MONICA Project populations. *Lancet*, 1999, **353**:1547–1557.

Table 3.1
Obesity prevalence (BMI ≥ 30) in some African countries and populations

Country or population	Year	Age (years)	Prevalence of obesity (%)		Reference
			Men	Women	
Ghana	1987–1988	20+	0.9		8
Mali	1991	20+	0.8		8
Mauritius	1992	25–74	5	15	7
Rodrigues (creoles)	1992	25–69	10	31	9
South Africa, Cape Peninsula (blacks)	1990	15–64	8	44	10
United Republic of Tanzania	1986–1989	35–64	0.6	3.6	11

it could be argued that Mauritius is not typical of other countries in the African Region, this study highlights both the adverse effects of lifestyle change in rapidly modernizing populations and how quickly obesity can become a public health problem.

3.4.2 *Current prevalence of obesity*

From the fragmentary and limited prevalence data available, it is evident that obesity does exist in the developing as well as in the more developed countries in the African Region, particularly among women. Table 3.1 shows data from a number of studies carried out in African countries.

In developing countries, rural adults still maintaining a traditional lifestyle gained little or no weight with age until relatively recently. This was formerly the case in Africa, and still is today in the few remaining hunter–gatherer populations, such as the San people, in northern Botswana (12). However, with the improvement in socio-economic status and increasing changes due to rapid urbanization, the prevalence of obesity among some groups of black women has risen markedly to levels exceeding those in populations in industrialized countries (13). In fact, approximately 44% of African women living in the Cape Peninsula were estimated to be obese in 1990 (10).

3.5 **Region of the Americas**

3.5.1 *Secular trends in obesity*

Secular trend data are available for Brazil, Canada and the USA, and are summarized in Table 3.2. These data indicate that obesity rates for both men and women are increasing not only in developed countries, but also in developing countries and in countries such as Brazil going through rapid socioeconomic transition.

Table 3.2
Trends in obesity (BMI ≥ 30) in selected countries in the Americas

Country	Year	Age (years)	Prevalence of obesity (%)		Reference
			Men	Women	
Brazil	1975	25–64	3.1	8.2	15
	1989	25–64	5.9	13.3	15
Canada	1978	20–70	6.8	9.6	16
	1981	20–70	8.5	9.3	17
	1988	20–70	9.0	9.2	18
	1986–1990	18–74	15.0	15.0	19
United States	1960–1962	20–74	10.4	15.1	14
of America	1971–1974	20–74	11.8	16.1	14
	1976–1980	20–74	12.3	16.5	14
	1988–1994	20–74	19.9	24.9	14

The most comprehensive data on national trends in the prevalence of obesity in a developed country in the Region are those for the USA. These are based on comparisons of data from NHES I (1960–1962), NHANES I (1971–1974), NHANES II (1976–1980), and NHANES III (1988–1994) (14). The figures for the USA presented in Table 3.2 are particularly valuable as they have been recalculated from those of the above-mentioned NHES and NHANES surveys for the WHO classification of obesity, i.e. BMI ≥ 30. These suggest that obesity is an escalating problem in the USA; there was a slight increase in the overall estimated prevalence of obesity during the period covered by the first three surveys, but a much larger increase between the third and the fourth surveys.

Data from Brazil provide the most valuable information on obesity prevalence and trends in a country in transition in the Region; two comparable, nationally representative, random nutrition surveys made 15 years apart make possible a detailed investigation of changing patterns of the nutritional status of children and adults, men and women, rich and poor. These surveys, which were undertaken by the Brazilian agency in charge of national statistics in 1974–1975 (the National Study of Family Expenditure (ENDEF) survey) and in 1989 (the National Survey on Health and Nutrition (PNSN)), show that adult obesity has increased in all groups of men and women. However, a greater increase has been observed among lower-income families. The problem of dietary deficit in Brazil is rapidly being replaced by one of dietary excess (15).

3.5.2 *Current prevalence of obesity*

The most recent data for the prevalence of obesity in the USA are those from NHANES III (1988–1994). A recent reanalysis of the data

Table 3.3
Obesity prevalence (BMI ≥ 30) in selected countries in the Americas

Country	Year	Age (years)	Prevalence of obesity (%) Men	Women	Reference
Brazil	1989	25–64	6	13	*15*
Canada	1986–1990	18–74	15.0	15.0	*19*
USA	1988–1994	20–74	19.9	24.9	*14*

using BMI ≥30 to classify obesity is particularly valuable for use in global comparisons, and showed that around 20% of all men and 25% of all women in the USA are obese. Table 3.3 shows that, in the early 1990s, obesity was more widespread in the USA than in Canada. Detailed subgroup analysis of the data shows that black women and other minority populations in the USA tend to have particularly high rates of obesity.

The only Latin American country to have conducted a nationally representative survey in the last 10 years is Brazil. The PNSN survey indicated that obesity is prevalent in Brazil, affecting about 6% of men and 13% of women in 1989 (*15*).

Evidence from the Caribbean, specifically Barbados, Cuba, Jamaica and Saint Lucia, indicates that obesity is a significant problem in this region. It is more common in those countries with a higher per capita GNP, affects women more than men, and is associated with a parallel increase in the prevalence of hypertension and NIDDM (*20*). However, as an unusual classification system (obese males: BMI ≥31.1; obese females: BMI ≥32.3) is used, the study is not cited in Table 3.3.

3.6 South-East Asia Region

3.6.1 *Secular trends in obesity*

Good-quality, nationally representative, secular trend data for countries in the South-East Asia Region were unavailable. However, data from two studies conducted by the same research centre in Thailand do suggest that diet-related chronic diseases, including obesity, are increasing in affluent urban populations. The first study was conducted in 1985 among 35–54-year-old Thai officials; it was found that 2.2% of the 2703 men, and 3.0% of the 792 women, had a BMI ≥30 (*21*). The second study in 1991 was smaller (66 men and 453 women), and had a broader age range (19–61 years), but also assessed nutritional factors in affluent urban Thais. Results of this study showed that 3.0% of men and 3.8% of women had a BMI ≥30. Prevalence figures for BMI 25–29.9 were considerably higher (15.2% in men and 23.2% in women) (22).

3.6.2 Current prevalence of obesity

Only limited obesity prevalence data are available for countries in the Region. Various studies on nutritional status have been carried out, particularly in India, but these have generally been on undernutrition and on selected population groups and have not used the WHO classification of obesity. As many countries in south-east Asia are currently going through the so-called "nutrition transition",[1] there is a special need to collect good-quality, nationally representative obesity prevalence data. The nutrition transition is associated with a change in the structure of the diet, reduced physical activity and rapid increases in the prevalence of obesity (23).

3.7 European Region

3.7.1 Secular trends in obesity

Although the most comprehensive data on the prevalence of obesity in Europe are those of the WHO MONICA study (2), the 42 popula-tions in 38 centres chosen across Europe are not necessarily represen-tative of their host countries, and only data from the first cycle have so far been published.[2] The best picture of secular trends in obesity prevalence in European countries should therefore be provided by data from national surveys. Population-level trend data on obesity prevalence in Europe are available for several countries, including England, Finland, Germany, the Netherlands and Sweden. Some of these data are summarized in Table 3.4, from which it can be seen that the prevalence of obesity has increased by about 10–40% in the majority of European countries in the past 10 years. The most dra-matic increase has been observed in England, where it has more than doubled during this period (24). There is some evidence, however, that there has been less of an increase among women in recent years, at least in some Scandinavian countries (25).

3.7.2 Current prevalence of obesity

Obesity is relatively common in Europe, especially among women and in southern and eastern European countries. The average preva-

---

[1] The rapid transition, or shift, from the problem of dietary deficit (or undernutrition) to one of dietary excess (or overnutrition and/or unbalanced nutrition).
[2] Updated material has been published since the Consultation: Tunstall-Pedoe H et al. Contribution of trends in survival and coronary-event rates to changes in coronary heart disease mortality: 10-year results from 37 WHO MONICA project populations. *Lancet*, 1999, 353:1547–1557.

Table 3.4
Trends in obesity (BMI ≥ 30) in selected European countries

Country	Year	Age (years)	Prevalence of obesity (%)		Reference
			Men	Women	
England	1980	16–64	6.0	8.0	*26*
	1986–1987		7	12	
	1991		12.7	15.0	
	1994		13.2	16.0	*27*
	1995		15.0	16.5	*24*
Finland	1978–1979	20–75	10	10	*28*
	1985–1987		12	10	
	1991–1993		14	11	
Former German	1985	25–65	13.7	22.2	L. Heinman,
Democratic	1989		13.4	20.6	personal
Republic	1992		20.5	26.8	communication,
					1996
Netherlands	1987	20–29	6.0	8.5	*29*
	1988		6.3	7.6	
	1989		6.2	7.4	
	1990		7.4	9.0	
	1991		7.5	8.8	
	1992		7.5	9.3	
	1993		7.1	9.1	
	1994		8.8	9.4	
	1995		8.4	8.3	
Sweden	1980–1981	16–84	4.9	8.7[a]	*30*
	1988–1989		5.3	9.1[a]	

[a] Obesity is defined as BMI >28.6.

lence of obesity in European centres participating in the WHO MONICA study between 1983 and 1986 was about 15% in men and 22% in women, although there was great variability both within and between countries. The lowest prevalence was found in Gothenburg, Sweden (men 7%, women 9%) and the highest in Kaunas, USSR (now Lithuania) (men 22%, women 45%).

The most recent data from individual national studies suggest that the prevalence of obesity in European countries is currently in the range 10–20% in men and 10–25% in women (Table 3.5). In agreement with the MONICA data, the prevalence of obesity is generally higher in women than in men.

3.8 Eastern Mediterranean Region

3.8.1 *Secular trends in obesity*

Good-quality, nationally representative, secular trend data for countries in the Eastern Mediterranean Region are not available.

Table 3.5
Obesity prevalence (BMI ≥ 30) in selected European countries

Country	Year	Age (years)	Prevalence of obesity (%)		Reference
			Men	Women	
Former Czechoslovakia	1988	20–65	16	20	V. Hainer, personal communication, 1997; *31*
England	1995	16–64	15	16.5	*24*
Finland	1991–1993	20–75	14	11	*28*
Former Federal Republic of Germany	1990	25–69	17	19	*32*
Former German Democratic Republic	1992	25–69	21	27	L. Heinman, personal communication, 1996
Netherlands	1995	20–59	8	8	*29*

3.8.2 *Current prevalence of obesity*

Data on the prevalence of adult obesity in the Eastern Mediterranean Region have not been well documented at the national level except in Saudi Arabia. Various surveys have been conducted but these have tended to be only for specific population groups within a country, such as women attending an infertility clinic, and/or have not classified obesity as BMI ≥30. Nevertheless, the limited data available, some of which are shown in Table 3.6, indicate that the prevalence of adult obesity in countries in the Region is high, and that women in particular are affected. In general, the prevalence of obesity among women is higher than that reported for women in most industrialized countries.

A nationally representative, cross-sectional survey was conducted between 1990 and 1993 to study the effects of sex, age and regional distribution on the prevalence of overweight and obesity among 13 177 randomly selected adult Saudi subjects. The prevalence of obesity among the female subjects was several-fold higher than the reported prevalence in more highly industrialized countries, and was higher than among male subjects for all regions of Saudi Arabia (*33*).

In the United Arab Emirates, obesity is recognized as a major public health problem that may play an important role in the increasing incidence of other chronic diseases. Data from the National Nutrition Survey showed that 38% of married women and 15.8% of married

Table 3.6
Obesity prevalence (BMI ≥ 30) in selected Eastern Mediterranean countries

Country	Year	Age (years)	Prevalence of obesity (%)		Reference
			Men	Women	
Bahrain:	1991–1992	20–65			35
Urban			9.5	30.3	
Rural			6.5	11.2	
Cyprus	1989–1990	35–64	19	24	13
Iran, Islamic Republic of (south)	1993–1994	20–74	2.5	7.7	36
Kuwait	1994	18+	32	41	37
Saudi Arabia:	1990–1993	15+			33
Total			16	24	
Urban			18	28	
Rural			12	18	
United Arab Emirates	1992	17+	16	38	34

men were obese (*34*). In Bahrain, obesity was more common in urban than in rural areas, especially in women (*35*).

Finally, a recent study in the south of the Islamic Republic of Iran revealed that obesity is prevalent in the adult population, and is more frequent among women than men (*36*).

3.9 Western Pacific Region

3.9.1 *Secular trends in obesity*

Trend data on the prevalence of overweight and obesity in countries in the Western Pacific Region are available for Australia, China, Japan and Samoa. These are summarized in Table 3.7 and show an increasing prevalence of obesity among Australians and Samoans. The Australian data are from three National Heart Foundation studies conducted in the six state capitals in 1980 and 1983, with two extra cities added in 1989 (*38*). Rural residents were not included.

Detailed analysis of data from the National Nutrition Survey in Japan conducted by the Japanese Ministry of Health and Welfare (*n* = 5000 per year) has shown that there has been a secular increase in obesity in both men and women during the period 1976–1993. Obesity among men increased by a factor of about 2.4; in women, in the 20–29-year age group, obesity increased by a factor of about 1.8 (S. Inoue, personal communication).

Table 3.7
Trends in obesity (BMI ≥ 30) in selected Western Pacific countries

Country	BMI cut-off	Year	Age (years)	Prevalence of obesity (%)		Reference
				Men	Women	
Australia		1980	25–64	9.3	8.0	*38*
		1983		9.1	10.5	
		1989		11.5	13.2	
China	27	1989	20–45	1.7	4.3	*39*
		1991		2.9	4.3	
	30	1989	20–45	0.29	0.89	C. Chunming,
		1991		0.36	0.86	personal
						communication
Japan	26.4	1976	20+	7.1	12.3	S. Inoue,
		1982		8.4	12.3	personal
		1987		10.3	12.6	communication
		1993		11.8	13.0	
	30	1976	20+	0.7	2.8	S. Inoue,
		1982		0.9	2.6	personal
		1987		1.3	2.8	communication
		1993		1.8	2.6	
Samoa:	30	1978	25–69	38.8	59.1	*40*
Urban		1991		58.4	76.8	
Rural	30	1978	25–69	17.7	37.0	*40*
		1991		41.5	59.2	

Data for 1989 and 1991 from the China Health and Nutrition Survey (CHNS) show an increase in the proportion of adult men, but not women, who are severely overweight (BMI ≥ 27) and obese (BMI ≥ 30) (*39*). This longitudinal survey, which is now under way, is considered to be representative of all provinces in China. As the plan is for surveys to be conducted every two years, the CHNS should prove a valuable source of data for documenting the secular trends in obesity in a country in economic transition. Data from the 1993 survey have been published since the time of the WHO Consultation.[1]

Secular trends have also been observed in Samoa, where there has been a marked increase in the prevalence of obesity between 1978

---

[1] Wang Y, Popkin B, Zhai F. The nutritional status and dietary pattern of Chinese adolescents, 1991 and 1993. *European Journal of Clinical Nutrition*, 1998, **52**(12):908–916.
Guo X et al. Food price policy can favorably alter macronutrient intake in China. *Journal of Nutrition*, 1999, **129**:994–1001.

and 1991, especially among men living in rural areas. Obesity is not new to Pacific populations and has long been regarded as attractive and a symbol of high social status and prosperity (40). However, there is evidence that these traditional notions are being replaced by an image of small body size (41).

3.9.2 Current prevalence of obesity

Table 3.8 shows the most recent estimates of obesity rates in a number of countries in the Western Pacific. The prevalence of obesity in the general population of both Australia and New Zealand appears to be in the range 10–15%. Studies of Aborigines living in different regions of Australia are not consistent with this finding; depending on the degree of "westernization" of Aboriginal communities, they have either a much higher or a substantially lower prevalence of obesity than the general Australian population (42).

Interim data from the Japanese National Nutrition Survey show that the prevalence of obesity in Japan is around 2% in males and 3% in females. When a BMI cut-off point of 26.4 is used (≥120% of standard body weight (SBW)), the figures are around 12% and 13%, respectively. Various studies have also been conducted on specific population groups and centres within Japan (S. Inoue, personal communication).

The current prevalence of obesity in China is probably best documented by the 1992 third Nationwide Nutritional Survey (NNS III). This survey was conducted throughout both urban and rural provinces, and data were collected from a larger representative sample of men ($n = 14\,964$) and women ($n = 14\,590$) aged 20–45 years than the CHNS cohort ($n = 5000$ approximately). Data from NNS III show that obesity does exist in China, albeit at a low prevalence, is more common in women than in men (Table 3.8), and is more prevalent in urban than in rural areas. These findings are supported by a study in 11 478 randomly selected Chinese adults aged 40 years and older, although slightly higher rates were reported than in the younger age group studied in NNS III (C. Chunming, personal communication). A number of other data sets are available but the WHO classification of obesity is rarely used in them, they are not age-standardized and tend not to be nationally representative.

The most striking feature of Table 3.8 is the extremely high age-standardized prevalence of obesity observed in the Pacific island populations of Melanesia, Micronesia and Polynesia. In urban Samoa, for example, the prevalence of obesity has been estimated to be over 75% in adult women and almost 60% in adult men. However,

Table 3.8
Obesity prevalence (BMI ≥ 30) in selected Western Pacific countries

Country	Year	Age (years)	Prevalence of obesity (%)		Reference
			Men	Women	
Australia	1989	25–64	11.5	13.2	*38*
China	1992	20–45	1.20	1.64	C. Chunming, personal communication
Japan	1993	20+	1.7	2.7	S. Inoue, personal communication
Nauru (Micronesia)	1987	25–69	64.8	70.3	*40*
New Zealand	1989	18–64	10	13	*43*
Papua New Guinea (Melanesia):	1991	25–69			*40*
Coastal urban			36.3	54.3	
Coastal rural			23.9	18.6	
Highlands			4.7	5.3	
Samoa (Polynesia):	1991	25–69			*40*
Urban			58.4	76.8	
Rural			41.5	59.2	

Swinburn et al. (*44*) recently concluded that Polynesians seem leaner than Caucasians at any given body size, so that the prevalence of obesity in Polynesian populations may not be quite as high as is currently estimated using Caucasian-derived classifications based on BMI. The prevalence in rural populations is also extremely high, but lower than in urban areas.

Among adults aged 18–60 years in Malaysia, 4.7% of men and 7.9% of women were found to have a BMI above 30. In the women, over-weight and obesity problems were more serious in the Indian popula-tion; 17.1% of Indian women had a BMI over 30 compared to 8.8% of Malay and 4.3% of Chinese women. Among the Malay population, a considerably higher proportion of both men and women had a BMI over 30 (men: 5.6% urban, 1.8% rural; women: 8.8% urban, 2.6% rural), whereas the reverse was true for undernutrition; prevalence rates of undernutrition for men and women were 7% and 11% in urban areas and 11% and 14% in rural areas, respectively. Overall, overweight (BMI ≥25) was more prevalent than undernutrition in both urban and rural settings (*45*).

3.10 Body mass index distribution in adult populations

BMI distribution varies significantly according to the stage of devel-opment reached in a transitional society. As the proportion of the

Figure 3.3
BMI distribution of various adult populations worldwide (both sexes)[a]

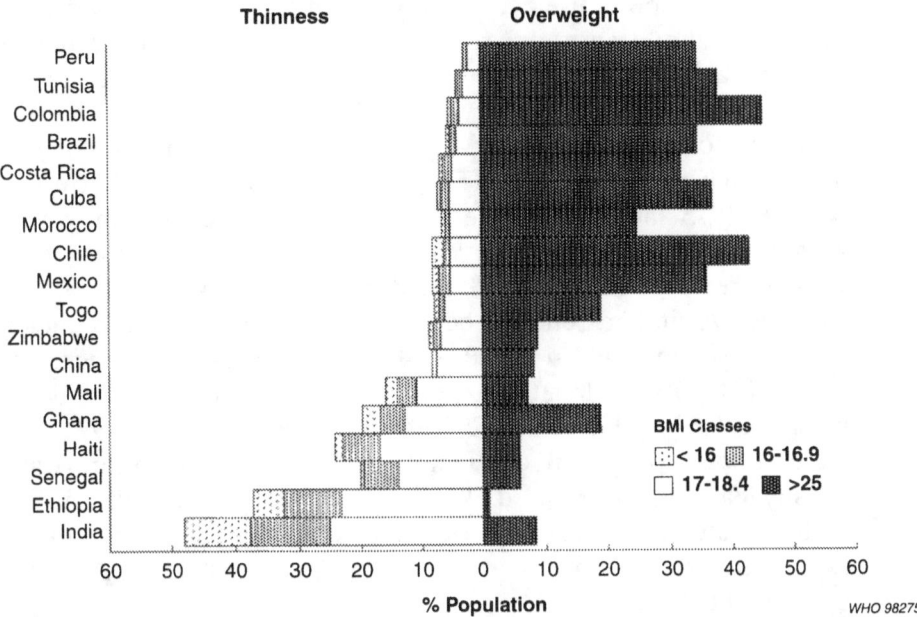

There is a tendency for an almost symmetrical increase in the proportion of a population with high BMI as the proportion of the population with low BMI decreases.

[a] Source: reference *11*.

population with a low BMI decreases, there is an almost symmetrical increase in the proportion with a BMI above 25 (Fig. 3.3). This indicates a tendency for a population-wide shift to take place as socio-economic conditions improve, with overweight replacing thinness.

In the first stages of the transition, the wealthier sections of society show an increase in the proportion of people with a high BMI, whereas thinness remains the main concern among the less wealthy. Thus, in countries in the early stage of transition, overweight can coexist with underweight, so that the burden of disease may be doubled.

The distribution of BMI tends to change again in the later phases of the transition, with an increase in the prevalence of high BMI among the poor.

3.11 Obesity during childhood and adolescence

The lack of consistency and agreement between different studies in the classification of obesity in children and adolescents (see section 2) means that it is not yet possible to give an overview of the global prevalence of obesity in these younger age groups. Nevertheless, whatever method is used to classify obesity, studies of this disease during childhood and adolescence have generally reported both a high prevalence and rates that are increasing. In the USA, for example, the prevalence of overweight (defined by the 85th percentile of weight-for-height) among 5–24-year-olds from a biracial community of Louisiana (total $n = 11\,564$) increased approximately twofold between 1973 and 1994. Furthermore, the yearly increases in relative weight and obesity during the latter part of the study period (1983–1994) were approximately 50% greater than those between 1973 and 1982 (*46*). A similar trend has been observed in Japan; the frequency of obese schoolchildren (>120% SBW) aged 6–14 years increased from 5% to 10%, and that of extremely obese (>140% SBW) children from 1% to 2% during the 20 years between 1974 and 1993. The increase was most prominent in male students aged 9–11 years. Early obesity leads to an increased likelihood of obesity in later life, as well as to an increased prevalence of obesity-related disorders. In the Japanese study, approximately one-third of obese children grew into obese adults (*47*).

Childhood obesity is not confined to the industrialized countries, as high rates are already evident in some developing countries. The prevalence of obesity among schoolchildren aged 6–12 years in Thailand, as diagnosed by weight-for-height exceeding 120% of the Bangkok reference, rose from 12.2% in 1991 to 15.6% in 1993 (*48*), and in a recent study of 6–18-year-old male schoolchildren in Saudi Arabia, the prevalence of obesity was found to be 15.8% (*49*).

The only integrated data currently available that give an overview of the global prevalence of obesity during childhood are those compiled by the WHO Programme of Nutrition (*50, 51*). In the WHO analysis, children were classified as obese when they exceeded the NCHS median weight-for-height plus two standard deviations or Z-scores.[1] The reported prevalence of obese children for the age group 0–4.99 years is shown in Fig. 3.4. It should be noted, however, that some children classified as obese under this system may actually have a higher relative weight due to stunting rather than as a result of excess adiposity. This is of particular significance in developing countries

---

[1] The Z-score is the deviation of an individual's value from the median value of a reference population divided by the standard deviation of the reference population.

Figure 3.4
Prevalence of obese preschool children (0–59 months) in selected countries and territories[a]

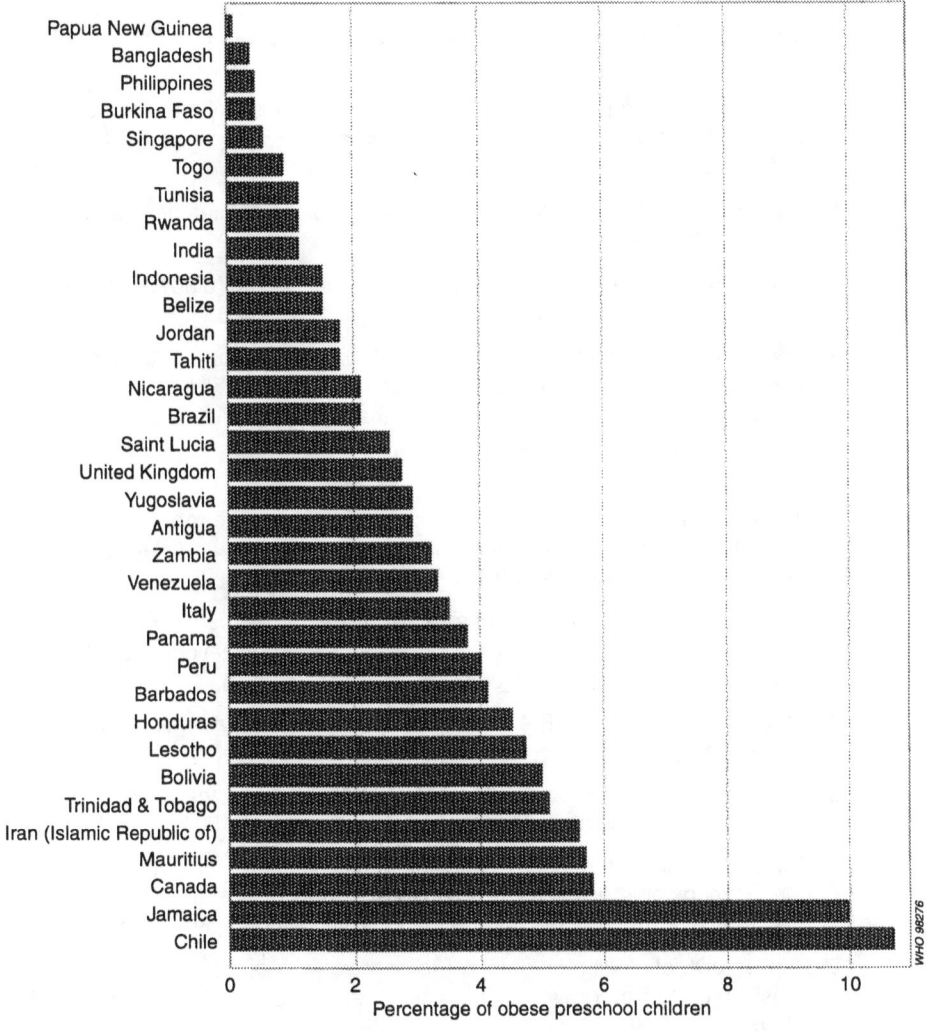

Obesity is defined as more than two standard deviations above the reference median weight-for-height (NCHS reference population).

[a] Source: reference *52*.

undergoing the nutrition transition, where a higher risk of obesity in stunted children has been described (*53*).

There is an urgent need to evaluate existing and future data sources concerning children and adolescents from across the world based on a standardized obesity classification system.

References

1. *World health statistics annual 1995.* Geneva, World Health Organization, 1996.

2. WHO MONICA Project: Risk Factors. *International Journal of Epidemiology,* 1989, 18(Suppl. 1):S46–S55.

3. WHO MONICA Project: Geographical variation in the major risk factors of coronary heart disease in men and women aged 35–64 years. *World Health Statistics Quarterly,* 1988, **41**:115–140.

4. **Chan JM et al.** Obesity, fat distribution, and weight gain as risk factors for clinical diabetes in men. *Diabetes Care,* 1994, **17**:961–969.

5. **Colditz GA et al.** Weight gain as a risk factor for clinical diabetes mellitus in women. *Annals of Internal Medicine,* 1995, **122**:481–486.

6. **Dowse GK et al.** Changes in population cholesterol concentrations and other cardiovascular risk factor levels after five years of the non-communicable disease intervention programme in Mauritius. *British Medical Journal,* 1995, **311**:1255–1259.

7. **Hodge AM et al.** Incidence, increasing prevalence, and predictors of change in obesity and fat distribution over 5 years in the rapidly developing population of Mauritius. *International Journal of Obesity and Related Metabolic Disorders,* 1996, **20**:137–146.

8. *Physical status: the use and interpretation of anthropometry. Report of a WHO Expert Committee.* Geneva, World Health Organization, 1995 (WHO Technical Report Series, No. 854).

9. **Hodge AM, Zimmet PZ.** The epidemiology of obesity. *Baillieres Clinical Endocrinology and Metabolism,* 1994, **8**:577–599.

10. **Steyn K et al.** Risk factors for coronary heart disease in the black population of the Cape Peninsula. *South African Medical Journal,* 1991, **79**:480–485.

11. **Berrios X et al.** Distribution and prevalence of major risk factors of noncommunicable diseases in selected countries: the WHO Inter-Health Programme. *Bulletin of the World Health Organization,* 1997, **75**:99–108.

12. **Hansen JDL et al.** Hunter–gatherer to pastoral way of life: effects of the transition on health, growth and nutritional status. *South African Journal of Science,* 1993, **89**:559–564.

13. **Walker ARP.** Epidemiology and health implications of obesity in Southern Africa. In: Fourie J, Steyn S, eds. *Chronic diseases of lifestyle in South Africa: review of research and identification of essential health research priority.* Cape Town, Medical Research Council, 1995, 73–85.

14. **Flegal KM et al.** Overweight and obesity in the United States: prevalence and trends, 1960–1994. *International Journal of Obesity,* 1998, **22**:39–47.

15. **Monteiro CA et al.** The nutrition transition in Brazil. *European Journal of Clinical Nutrition,* 1995, **49**:105–113.

16. **Health and Welfare Canada.** *The health of Canadians: report of the Canada Health Survey.* Ottawa, Ministry of Supplies and Services, Government of Canada, 1981.

17. *Canadian standardized test of fitness: operations manual*, 3rd ed. Ottawa, Fitness Canada, 1986.

18. Stephens T, Craig CL. *The well-being of Canadians: highlights of the 1988 Campbell's Survey*, Ottawa, Canadian Fitness and Lifestyle Research Institute, 1990.

19. Reeder BA et al. Obesity and its relation to cardiovascular disease risk factors in Canadian adults. *Canadian Medical Association Journal*, 1992, **146**:2009–2019.

20. Forrester T et al. Obesity in the Caribbean. In: Chadwick DJ, Cardeau G, eds. *The origins and consequences of obesity*. Chichester, Wiley, 1996:17–31.

21. Tanphaichitr V et al. Prevalence of obesity and its associated risks in urban Thais. In: Oomura Y et al., eds. *Progress in obesity research*, London, John Libbey, 1990:649–653.

22. Leelahagul P, Tanphaichitr V. Current status on diet-related chronic diseases in Thailand. *Internal Medicine*, 1995, **11**:28–33.

23. Popkin BM. The nutrition transition in low-income countries: an emerging crisis. *Nutrition Reviews*, 1994, **52**:285–298.

24. Prescott-Clarke P, Primatesta P. *Health survey for England 1995*. London, Her Majesty's Stationery Office, 1997.

25. Pietinen P, Vartiainen E, Männistö S. Trends in body mass index and obesity among adults in Finland from 1972 to 1992. *International Journal of Obesity and Related Metabolic Disorders*, 1996, **20**:114–120.

26. *Obesity: reversing the increasing problem of obesity in England. A report from the Nutrition and Physical Activity Task Forces*. London, Department of Health, 1995.

27. Colhoun H, Prescott-Clarke P. *Health survey for England 1994*. London, Her Majesty's Stationery Office, 1996.

28. Seidell JC, Rissanen AM. Time trends in the worldwide prevalence of obesity. In: Bray GA, Bouchard C, James WPT, eds. *Handbook of obesity*. New York, Marcel Dekker, 1998:79–91.

29. Seidell JC. Time trends in obesity: an epidemiological perspective. *Hormone and Metabolic Research*, 1997, **29**:155–158.

30. Kuskowska-Wolk A, Bergström R. Trends in body mass index and prevalence of obesity in Swedish women 1980–89. *Journal of Epidemiology and Community Health*, 1993, **47**:195–199.

31. Hainiš K, Petrásek R. Body height, weight and BMI for the Czech and Slovak populations. *Homo*, 1999, **52**:163–182.

32. Hoffmeister H, Mensink GBM, Stolzenberg H. National trends in risk factors for cardiovascular diseases in Germany. *Preventive Medicine*, 1994, **23**:197–205.

33. Al-Nuaim A et al. Prevalence of diabetes mellitus, obesity and hypercholesterolemia in Saudi Arabia. In: Musaiger AO, Miladi SS, eds. *Diet-related non-communicable diseases in the Arab countries of the Gulf*. Cairo, Food and Agriculture Organization of the United Nations, 1996:73–81.

34. **Musaiger AO.** Trends in diet-related chronic diseases in United Arab Emirates. In: Musaiger AO, Miladi SS, eds. *Diet-related non-communicable diseases in the Arab countries of the Gulf.* Cairo, Food and Agriculture Organization of the United Nations, 1996:99–117.

35. **Al-Mannai A et al.** Obesity in Bahraini adults. *Journal of the Royal Society of Health*, 1996, **116**:30–40.

36. **Pishdad GR.** Overweight and obesity in adults aged 20–74 in southern Iran. *International Journal of Obesity and Related Metabolic Disorders*, 1996, **20**:963–965.

37. **Al-Isa AN.** Prevalence of obesity among adult Kuwaitis: a cross-sectional study. *International Journal of Obesity and Related Metabolic Disorders*, 1995, **19**:431–433.

38. **Bennett SA, Magnus P.** Trends in cardiovascular risk factors in Australia. Results from the National Heart Foundation's Risk Factor Prevalence Study, 1980–1989. *Medical Journal of Australia*, 1994, **161**:519–527.

39. **Popkin BM et al.** Body weight patterns among the Chinese: results from the 1989 and 1991 China Health and Nutrition Surveys. *American Journal of Public Health*, 1995, **85**:690–694.

40. **Hodge AM et al.** Prevalence and secular trends in obesity in Pacific and Indian Ocean island populations. *Obesity Research*, 1995, 3(Suppl. 2):77s–87s.

41. **Craig PL et al.** Do Polynesians still believe that big is beautiful? Comparison of body size perceptions and preferences of Cook Islands, Maori and Australians. *New Zealand Medical Journal*, 1996, **109**:200–203.

42. National Health and Medical Research Council (NHMRC). *Acting on Australia's weight: a strategic plan for the prevention of overweight and obesity.* Canberra, Australian Government Publishing Service, 1997.

43. **Ball MJ et al.** Obesity and body fat distribution in New Zealanders: a pattern of coronary heart disease risk. *New Zealand Medical Journal*, 1993, **106**:69–72.

44. **Swinburn BA et al.** Body composition differences between Polynesians and Caucasians assessed by bioelectrical impedance. *International Journal of Obesity and Related Metabolic Disorders*, 1996, **20**:889–894.

45. **Ismail MN et al.** Prevalence of obesity and chronic energy deficiency (CED) in adult Malaysians. *Malaysian Journal of Nutrition*, 1995, **1**:1–10.

46. **Freedman DS et al.** Secular increases in relative weight and adiposity among children over two decades: the Bogalusa Heart Study. *Pediatrics*, 1997, **99**:420–426.

47. **Kotani K et al.** Two decades of annual medical examinations in Japanese obese children: do obese children grow into obese adults? *International Journal of Obesity and Related Metabolic Disorders*, 1997, **21**:912–921.

48. **Mo-suwan L, Junjuna C, Puetpaiboon A.** Increasing obesity in school children in a transitional society and the effect of the weight control program. *Southeast Asian Journal of Tropical Medicine and Public Health*, 1993, **24**:590–594.

49. **al-Nuaim AR, Bamgboye EA, al-Herbish A.** The pattern of growth and obesity in Saudi Arabian male school children. *International Journal of Obesity and Related Metabolic Disorders*, 1996, **20**:1000–1005.

50. *Diet, nutrition and the prevention of chronic diseases. Report of a WHO Study Group.* Geneva, World Health Organization, 1990 (WHO Technical Report Series, No. 797).

51. WHO Global Database on Child Growth and Malnutrition. Geneva, World Health Organization, 1997 (unpublished document WHO/NUT/97.4, available on request from Department of Nutrition for Health and Development, World Health Organization, 1211 Geneva 27, Switzerland).

52. **Gurney M, Gorstein J.** The global prevalence of obesity — an initial overview of available data. *World Health Statistics Quarterly*, 1988, **41**:251–254.

53. **Popkin BM, Richards MK, Monteiro CA.** Stunting is associated with overweight in children of four nations that are undergoing the nutrition transition. *Journal of Nutrition*, 1996, **126**:3009–3016.

Establishing the true costs of the problem of overweight and obesity

4. Health consequences of overweight and obesity in adults and children

4.1 Introduction

The health consequences of obesity are many and varied, ranging from an increased risk of premature death to several non-fatal but debilitating complaints that have an adverse effect on quality of life. Obesity is also a major risk factor for NCDs such as NIDDM, CVD and cancer, and in many industrialized countries is associated with various psychosocial problems. Abdominal obesity is of particular concern as it is associated with greater risks to health than is a more peripheral fat distribution.

The health consequences of overweight and obesity in both adults and children are considered here, while the effect of weight loss on these conditions is discussed in section 5.

The key issues covered are:

- The major health consequences associated with overweight and obesity, namely NIDDM, CHD, hypertension, gallbladder disease, psychosocial problems and certain types of cancer.

- The lack of detailed relative risk data for the various health problems associated with obesity. These are available only for a few industrialized countries, and show that the risks of suffering from NIDDM, gallbladder disease, dyslipidaemia, insulin resistance and sleep apnoea are greatly increased in the obese (relative risk (RR) much greater than 3). The risks of CHD and osteoarthritis are moderately increased (RR 2–3) and the risks of certain cancers, reproductive hormone abnormalities and low back pain are slightly increased (RR 1–2).

- Biases such as failure to control for cigarette smoking and unintentional weight loss. When these are removed from the analysis of mortality data, there is an almost linear relationship between BMI and death. The longer the duration of obesity, the higher the risk. Severe obesity is associated with a 12-fold increase in mortality in 25–35-year-olds compared with lean individuals. This highlights the importance of preventing weight gain throughout adult life.

- Excess abdominal fat. This is an independent predictor for NIDDM, CHD, hypertension, breast cancer and premature death.

- Weight gain during early adulthood. Most of this is body fat, which increases health risks.

- The many non-fatal but debilitating conditions that affect the obese. These are responsible for a much reduced quality of life in overweight patients and are often the primary reason for contact with the health care system. Most of these conditions can be improved with modest weight loss.

- The psychosocial consequences of obesity. These have important implications for disease management, and are compounded by the fact that health professionals often view obese individuals as weak-willed and unlikely to benefit from counselling.

- The association between obesity and certain psychosocial consequences in adolescence, and the persistence of obesity into adulthood.

4.2 Obesity as a risk factor for noncommunicable diseases

Although obesity should be considered as a disease in its own right, it is also one of the key risk factors for other NCDs, such as NIDDM and CHD, together with smoking, high blood pressure and hypercholesterolaemia (1). The adverse health consequences of obesity are influenced to a greater or lesser extent by body weight, the location of body fat, the magnitude of weight gain during adulthood, and a sedentary lifestyle (2).

As a chronic disease, obesity has many similarities to hypertension and hypercholesterolaemia. Fig. 4.1 shows the positive relationship between relative risk of mortality and: (a) BMI (as an index of obesity); (b) cholesterol; and (c) diastolic blood pressure. In the "moderate-risk" category, which corresponds to the ranges between widely accepted cut-off points for lower and higher risk levels, an increase in any of the three variables greatly increases the risk of mortality. The increase is even steeper in the "high-risk" category, implying greater individual risk. However, from a population perspective, the middle range is of most concern as this encompasses the greatest number of people (2).

4.3 Difficulties in evaluating the health consequences of obesity

Most of the evidence linking health problems with obesity comes from prospective and cross-sectional population-based studies, although there is additional information from community interventions and clinical trials. Some confusion over the consequences of excess weight may arise because studies have used different BMI cut-off points for defining obesity, and because the presence of many medical conditions involved in the development of obesity may confound the effects of obesity itself.

Specific problems in evaluating the health consequences of obesity include:

Figure 4.1

**Relationship between (a) BMI, (b) cholesterol and (c) diastolic blood pressure
and relative risk of mortality[a]**

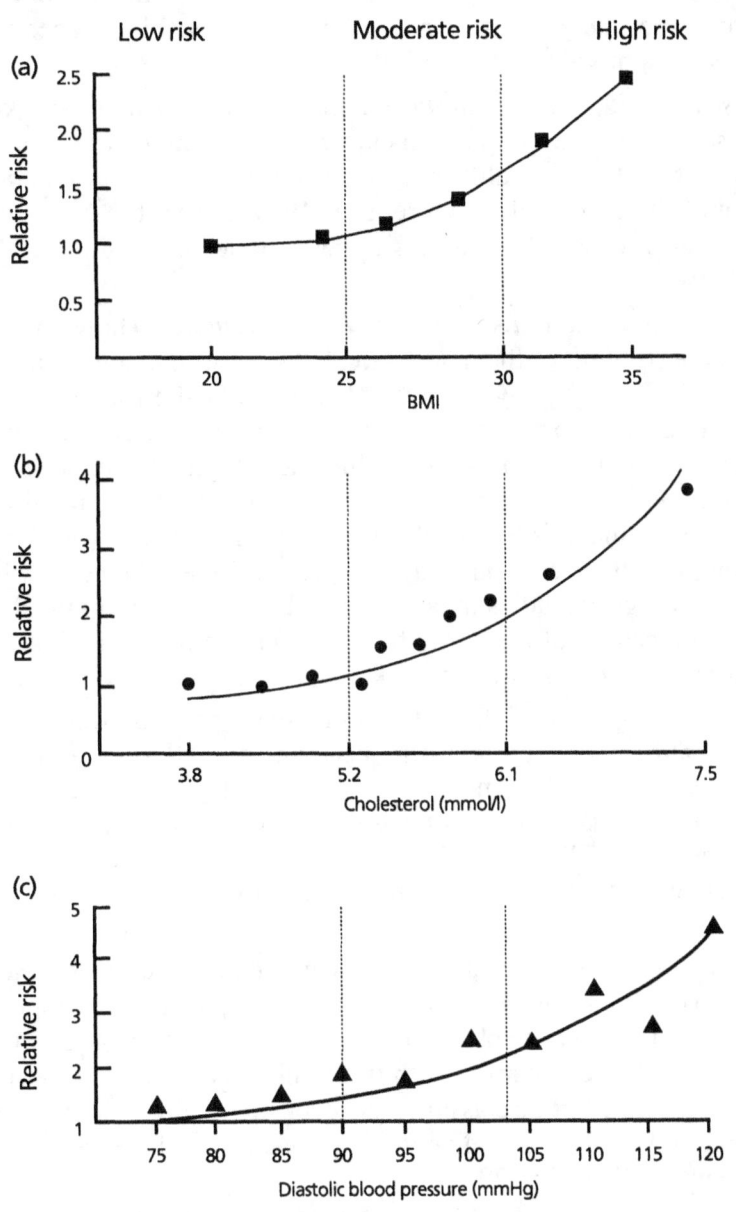

[a] Adapted from reference 2 with the permission of the publisher. Copyright John Wiley & Sons
Ltd. Based on data from Stamler et al. (3, 4) for the construction of the blood pressure and
cholesterol plots, and from the Nurses' Health Study (5) for the BMI plot. There are similar
continuous graded increases in the RR of mortality as BMI, blood pressure and cholesterol
increase. However, the RR rises more rapidly for cholesterol and blood pressure than it does
for BMI. The rise in the RR of mortality is notably steeper from BMI >30, cholesterol >6 mmol/
litre, and diastolic blood pressure >100 mmHg (13.3 kPa).

- *The continuous relationship between gradations of excess weight and morbidity.* Individuals who have gained weight but still lie within the normal range will be assigned to a normal weight category even though they may be at increased risk of comorbidity because of excess weight gain.

- *Present health status and health behaviours (such as smoking).* These may have an impact on current weight and confuse its association with future health or even current well-being. For example, smoking is associated with a reduced BMI, so that the incidence of lung cancer caused by smoking appears to decrease with increased body weight.

- *The duration and design of epidemiological studies.* These will influence the strength of the association between weight and morbidity. Long-term monitoring is required to identify the range of health consequences of obesity, whereas studies of shorter duration with a large study population can be useful in identifying the major impact of obesity. Longer-term studies are also required where the outcome, e.g. cancer, is the result of a multistage process, with obesity having an effect on some but not necessarily all the stages. Most epidemiological studies measure prevalence rather than incidence, with the result that they are often confounded by survival bias and post-morbid modification of risk.

- *The age group studied.* This affects the relationship between obesity and health. For example, if the incidence of CHD in men is being analysed, obesity is a much more important predictor at younger than at older ages. The reverse is true, however, if total mortality is the end-point. The reason for this may be that obesity at an earlier age affects intervening risk factors much more strongly than in later life.

- *The use of initial weight criteria.* Most epidemiological studies adopt (by necessity) a static approach to classifying people by weight, i.e. subjects are generally placed in a weight group at the beginning of the study. The association with future illness or events is therefore based on that initial classification even if weight is subsequently gained or lost. This may give the impression that there is a risk-free zone up to BMI 27 or 28, which is misleading; weight gain independent of BMI is an important risk factor, as is the distribution of the fat gained.

4.4 Relative risk of obesity-associated health problems

The non-fatal but debilitating health problems associated with obesity include respiratory difficulties, chronic musculoskeletal problems, skin problems and infertility.

Table 4.1
Relative risk of health problems associated with obesity[a]

Greatly increased (relative risk much greater than 3)	Moderately increased (relative risk 2–3)	Slightly increased (relative risk 1–2)
NIDDM	CHD	Cancer (breast cancer in postmenopausal women, endometrial cancer, colon cancer)
Gallbladder disease	Hypertension	Reproductive hormone abnormalities
Dyslipidaemia	Osteoarthritis (knees)	Polycystic ovary syndrome
Insulin resistance	Hyperuricaemia and gout	Impaired fertility
Breathlessness		Low back pain due to obesity
Sleep apnoea		Increased risk of anaesthesia complications
		Fetal defects associated with maternal obesity

[a] All relative risk values are approximate.

The more life-threatening, chronic health problems associated with obesity fall into four main areas: (a) cardiovascular problems, including hypertension, stroke and CHD; (b) conditions associated with insulin resistance, e.g. NIDDM; (c) certain types of cancers, especially the hormonally related and large-bowel cancers; and (d) gallbladder disease.

It is important to recognize that ethnic differences have a bearing on the prevalence of a particular disease; some minority populations in the USA have a higher prevalence of certain obesity-related diseases (particularly NIDDM but, for black Americans, also CVD, stroke and osteoarthritis of the knee) compared with the white population (6). Nevertheless, although the absolute prevalence may vary, the relative risk of any particular disease (i.e. whether the risk is slightly, moderately or greatly increased for an obese person as compared with a lean person) is fairly similar throughout the world (Table 4.1).

4.5 Intra-abdominal (central) fat accumulation and increased risk

Compared with subcutaneous adipose tissue, intra-abdominal adipose tissue has:

— more cells per unit mass;
— higher blood flow;
— more glucocorticoid (cortisol) receptors;

— probably more androgen (testosterone) receptors;
— greater catecholamine-induced lipolysis.

These differences make intra-abdominal adipose tissue more susceptible to both hormonal stimulation and changes in lipid accumulation
and metabolism. Furthermore, intra-abdominal adipocytes are
located upstream from the liver in the portal circulation. This means
that there is a marked increase in the flux of nonesterified fatty acid
(NEFA) to the liver via the portal blood in patients with abdominal
obesity.

There is good evidence that abdominal obesity is important in the
development of insulin resistance (see section 4.8.1), and in the metabolic syndrome (hyperinsulinaemia, dyslipidaemia, glucose intolerance, hypertension) that links obesity with CHD (see section 4.8.2).
Some non-Caucasian populations appear to be especially susceptible
to this type of syndrome, in which lifestyle changes may play a particularly important etiological role (7).

Premenopausal women have quantitatively more lipoprotein lipase
(LPL) and higher LPL activity in the gluteal and femoral subcutaneous regions, which contain fat cells larger than those in men, but
these differences disappear after the menopause (8). In contrast,
men show minimal regional variations in LPL activity or fat cell size.
These differences may explain the tendency for premenopausal
women to deposit fat preferentially in lower body fat depots. The
higher level of intra-abdominal adipose tissue found in men compared with premenopausal women seems to explain, in part, the
greater prevalence of dyslipidaemia and CHD in men than in premenopausal women.

4.6 Obesity-related mortality

There has been much controversy about the relationship between
obesity and mortality. While a number of studies have found a U- or
J-shaped association, with higher mortality rates at both the upper
and lower weight ranges, some have shown a gradual increase in
mortality with increasing weight, while others have reported no association at all.

Many studies relating obesity and mortality have included biases in
their design that have led to a systematic underestimate of the impact
of obesity on premature mortality. These include the failure to control for cigarette smoking (producing an artificially high mortality in
leaner subjects), inappropriate control for conditions such as hypertension and hyperglycaemia, which were assumed to be confounding

Figure 4.2
Relationship between BMI and relative risk of premature mortality[a]

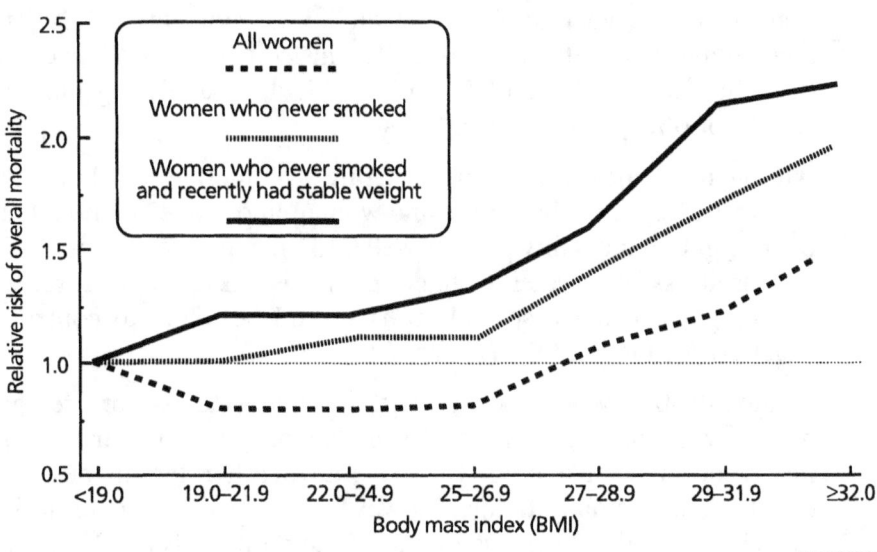

WHO 98285

The relationship between BMI and all-cause mortality was examined using data from the Nurses' Health Study, which involved 115 195 middle-aged women. A total of 4726 deaths occurred during the 16-year follow-up. The apparent excess relative risks of mortality associated with leanness, suggested when the analysis included all women, were found to be artefacts as they were eliminated by accounting for smoking (leaving 1499 deaths) and subclinical disease (leaving 531 deaths). By excluding former and current smokers, women with BMI < 22 were found to have the lowest mortality among the remaining women. When disease-related health loss was also accounted for, the leanest women (BMI < 19) had the lowest mortality. This analysis is based on professional middle-aged women and so may not be representative of all population groups.

[a] Based on data from Manson et al. (5), with permission, and reproduced from Gill PG, Key issues in the prevention of obesity, *British Medical Bulletin*, 1997, 53:359–388, with the permission of the publisher, Churchill Livingstone.

factors but are to a large degree the effects of obesity (hence some factorial analyses distort the true association between obesity and mortality), failure to control for weight loss associated with illness (leading to an underestimate of the impact of obesity on mortality), and failure to standardize for age (9, 10).

The Nurses' Health Study (5) in the USA found that, when biases are removed from the analysis, an almost linear, continuous relationship between BMI and mortality is found, with no specific lower threshold (see Fig. 4.2). This is not surprising, given the largely linear relationship between body weight and conditions such as CHD, hypertension and NIDDM when BMI increases from 20 to 30 (11–13). Similar results and conclusions have been reached by others (10, 14) but a follow-up study of NHANES has continued to show U-shaped curves after control of the pertinent variables. Nevertheless, whatever the shape of the curve, it appears that the lowest mortality risk is associated with a BMI between 18 and 25. This conclusion was reached by the American Institute of Nutrition (15) after analysing numerous studies of obesity and mortality risk.

Although the increase in mortality rate with increased relative body weight is steeper for both men and women under age 50, the effect of overweight on mortality persists well into the ninth decade of life. The increased risk observed in younger people is linked to the duration of overweight, so that a special effort should be made to control the weight of younger adults (14, 16, 17).

Finally, if obesity is associated with an increased risk of premature mortality, it may seem paradoxical that obesity rates are rising in many countries at a time when overall death rates in these same countries are actually falling. However, the decline in overall death rates is essentially the consequence of the reductions in CVD. These, in turn, are the result largely of falling rates of smoking and the improvement in dietary quality (higher intake of fruits and vegetables and reduced intake of salt, saturated fat and cholesterol). The incidence of NIDDM, however, is increasing, and there is evidence that this is a consequence of the rise in the prevalence of obesity. Increased obesity cannot be completely explained by reduced rates of smoking, which appear to be associated with only small increases in the average body weight of the population. The expected effect over time is an increase in mean BMI worldwide that will lead to a further increase in NIDDM, gallbladder disease, hypertension and atherosclerosis. Although these effects may not be reflected in overall mortality rate figures, they will surely lead to a higher frequency of the debilitating and prolonged morbidity from NCDs that require expensive health care.

4.7 Chronic diseases associated with obesity

4.7.1 Cardiovascular disease and hypertension

Cardiovascular disease
CVD encompasses CHD, stroke and peripheral vascular disease. CHD and stroke account for a large proportion of deaths in men and women in most industrialized countries, and their incidence is increasing in developing countries.

Obesity predisposes an individual to a number of cardiovascular risk factors including hypertension, raised cholesterol and impaired glucose tolerance. However, longer-term prospective data now suggest that obesity is also important as an independent risk factor for CHD-related morbidity and mortality (18). The Framingham Heart Study ranked body weight as the third most important predictor of CHD among males, after age and dyslipidaemia (19). Similarly, in women, a large-scale prospective study in the USA found a positive correlation between BMI and the risk of developing CHD. Weight gain substantially increased this risk (20). These findings are consistent with data from other countries. A 15-year follow-up study of 16000 men and women in eastern Finland concluded that obesity is an independent risk factor for CHD mortality in men and contributes to the risk of CHD in women (21).

On the basis of the Framingham Heart Study and other studies, it can be concluded that the degree of overweight is related to the rate of development of CVD (22). The CHD risk associated with obesity is higher in younger age groups and also in people with abdominal obesity than in those with excess fat around the hips and thighs (23) (see section 4.5). In addition, mortality from CHD has been shown to be increased in overweight individuals, even at body weights only 10% above the average (24).

Interestingly, Asian Indians have the highest rates of CHD of any ethnic group studied, despite the fact that nearly half this group are lifelong vegetarians. CHD occurs at an early age and generally follows a severe and progressive course. Although the prevalence of classic risk factors is relatively low, there is a substantial prevalence in this population of high triglyceride and low high-density lipoprotein (HDL) cholesterol levels, high lipoprotein (a) levels, hyperinsulinaemia and abdominal obesity (25). These appear to constitute weight-related risk factors in this population that may, in particular, reflect the central distribution of body fat.

Hypertension and stroke
The association between hypertension and obesity is well documented. Both systolic and diastolic blood pressure increase with BMI, and the obese are at higher risk of developing hypertension than lean individuals (4, 26). Community-wide surveys in the USA (NHANES II) show that the prevalence of hypertension in overweight adults is 2.9-fold higher than that for non-overweight adults (27). The risk in those aged 20–44 years is 5.6 times greater than that in those aged 45–74 years (28), which in turn is twice as high as that for non-overweight adults (29). The risk of developing hypertension increases with the duration of obesity, especially in women, and weight reduction leads to a fall in blood pressure (see section 5.3.1).

A 1.00 kPa (7.5 mmHg) difference in diastolic pressure within the range 70–110 mmHg (9.33–14.7 kPa) is accompanied by a 29% difference in CHD risk and a 46% difference in the risk of stroke, irrespective of sex, age group or ethnicity (30).

While many large studies have examined the relationship between obesity and CHD, there has not been the same emphasis on stroke. One study in Honolulu, in which 1163 non-smoking men aged between 55 and 68 years were examined, found that elevated BMI was associated with increased risk of thromboembolic stroke (31). However, preliminary results obtained from women in the Swedish Obese Subjects (SOS) study were not conclusive (32). Other studies found that a high WHR rather than BMI was the risk factor associated with stroke and that this relationship was stronger than for any other anthropometric variable tested (33, 34). It was suggested that a lifelong history of obesity rather than weight in middle age is more important in assessing risk of stroke (13).

The reason for the association between increased body weight and elevated blood pressure is unclear. One possibility is that obesity is associated with higher circulating levels of insulin (a consequence of insulin resistance) and consequently with enhanced renal retention of sodium, resulting in increased blood pressure (35). As exercise is known to improve insulin sensitivity, this would perhaps explain why exercise also reduces blood pressure. Other possible etiological factors include elevated plasma renin or enhanced catecholamine activity (36).

4.7.2 Cancer

A number of studies have found a positive association between overweight and the incidence of cancer, particularly of hormone-dependent and gastrointestinal cancers (Table 4.2).

Greater risks of endometrial, ovarian, cervical and postmenopausal breast cancer have been documented for obese women, while there is some evidence for an increased risk of prostate cancer among obese men. The increased incidence of these cancers in the obese is greater in those with excess abdominal fat and is thought to be a direct consequence of hormonal changes (37). The incidence of gastrointestinal cancers, such as colorectal and gallbladder cancer, has also been reported to be positively associated with body weight or obesity in some but not all studies, and renal cell cancer has consistently been associated with overweight and obesity, especially in women (38, 39).

In addition to overall obesity, intra-abdominal fat distribution and adult weight gain have been independently associated with an

Table 4.2
Cancers with a higher reported incidence in obese persons

Hormone-dependent	Gastrointestinal/hepatic/renal
Endometrial	Colorectal
Ovarian	Gallbladder
Breast	Pancreatic
Cervical	Hepatic
Prostate	Renal

increased risk of breast cancer. For example, it has been reported that an increase in intra-abdominal fat accumulation increases the risk of postmenopausal breast cancer, independently of relative weight and particularly when there is a family history of the disease. Furthermore, weight gain during adulthood has consistently been associated with increased risk of breast cancer, even in cohort studies that showed no association between baseline relative weight and subsequent risk of breast cancer (*40, 41*).

In one major prospective study, in which 750 000 men and women were followed for 12 years, it was found that the mortality ratios[1] for any cancer were 1.33 and 1.55 for obese men and women, respectively (*42*). It should be noted, however, that in some studies of gastrointestinal and breast cancer, it has been difficult to determine whether it is the effect of dietary components that promote weight gain, such as a high fat content, or the effect of obesity per se that is important. Further research in this area is necessary.

High levels of physical activity have been shown to decrease the risk of colon cancer in men in the majority of studies, and in women in half the studies. However, the effect of physical activity on rectal cancer was not significant in most cases. Breast cancer and cancers of the reproductive system were less prevalent in women who had been athletes at college (*43*) compared with less active women. NHANES I data indicate that a high level of non-recreational activity is important in reducing the risk of cancer, but that there is only a weak relationship between recreational exercise and cancer, with the exception of prostate cancer (*44*).

4.7.3 *Diabetes mellitus*

A positive association between obesity and the risk of developing NIDDM has been repeatedly observed in both cross-sectional

---

[1] Ratio of premature deaths (<65 years) in a population with BMI ≥30 to premature deaths in a population with BMI <25.

(45–57) and prospective studies (53, 58–66). The consistency of the association across populations despite different measures of fatness and criteria for diagnosing NIDDM reflects the strength of the relationship. When women aged 30–55 years were monitored for 14 years, the additional risk of developing NIDDM for those who were obese was over 40 times greater than for women who remained slim (BMI <22) (61). The risk of NIDDM increases continuously with BMI and decreases with weight loss. Analysis of data from two recent large prospective studies illustrates the impact of overweight and obesity on NIDDM; about 64% of male and 74% of female cases of NIDDM could theoretically have been prevented if no one had had a BMI over 25 (61, 66).

Detailed analyses of the relationship between obesity and NIDDM have identified certain characteristics of obese persons that further increase the risk of developing this condition, even after controlling for age, smoking and family history of NIDDM. These include obesity during childhood and adolescence, progressive weight gain from 18 years, and intra-abdominal fat accumulation. In particular, intra-abdominal fat accumulation has been implicated as an independent risk factor for NIDDM in a variety of populations and ethnic groups around the world and, in some studies, has been an even stronger predictor of NIDDM than overall fatness (52, 56, 60).

Lack of physical activity and an unhealthy diet, both of which are associated with lifestyle in industrialized countries, are also important modifiable risk factors for overweight and obesity. The prevalence of NIDDM is 2–4-fold higher in the least physically active individuals compared with the most physically active (67, 68), an effect which is independent of the level of body mass, and a healthy diet can reverse the deterioration in glucose tolerance commonly seen with diets high in fat and low in carbohydrate and fibre (69).

Intra-abdominal fat accumulation, as well as obesity per se, are also associated with an increase in the risk of prediabetic conditions such as impaired glucose tolerance and insulin resistance. The benefits of weight loss in controlling NIDDM are discussed in section 5.

4.7.4 *Gallbladder disease*

In the general population, gallstones are more common in women and the elderly. However, obesity is a risk factor for gallstones in all age groups and, in both men and women, gallstones occur three to four times more often in obese compared with non-obese individuals, and the risk is even greater when excess fat is located around the abdomen. The relative risk of gallstones increases with BMI, and data from the Nurses' Health Study suggest that even moderate overweight may increase the risk (70).

Supersaturation of the bile with cholesterol and reduced motility of the gallbladder, both of which are present in the obese, are thought to be factors underlying gallstone formation. Furthermore, since gallstones enhance the propensity to gallbladder inflammation, acute and chronic cholecystitis is also more common in the obese. Biliary colic and acute pancreatitis are other potential complications of gallstones.

Paradoxically, gallstones are also a common clinical problem in those losing weight (see section 5).

4.8 Endocrine and metabolic disturbances associated with obesity

4.8.1 *Endocrine disturbances*

Recent research has shown that adipocytes (fat cells) are more than just fat depots. They also function as endocrine cells, producing many locally and distantly acting hormones, and as target cells for a great many hormones. Altered hormonal patterns have been observed in obese patients, especially in those with intra-abdominal fat accumulation (71, 72). Common hormonal abnormalities associated with intra-abdominal fat accumulation are listed in Table 4.3.

Insulin resistance

Sensitivity to insulin varies widely among any group of people, but insulin resistance is very often associated with obesity. It is especially pronounced with intra-abdominal fat accumulation and, since abdominal fat mass increases with increasing adiposity, is universally found in very severe obesity (BMI ≥40).

It has been suggested by some investigators that insulin resistance is an adaptation to obesity that tends to limit further fat deposition (73). In insulin resistance, the oxidation of fat tends to be favoured rather than its storage and the oxidation of glucose. Thus, if an individual

Table 4.3

Common hormonal abnormalities associated with intra-abdominal fat accumulation

Insulin resistance and increased insulin secretion
Increased free testosterone and free androstenedione levels associated with
  decreased sex hormone binding globulin (SHBG) in women
Decreased progesterone levels in women
Decreased testosterone levels in men
Increased cortisol production
Decreased growth hormone levels

who is gaining weight continues to eat the same amount, there will come a time at which net fat oxidation will, through insulin resistance, equal dietary fat intake and the individual will be in fat balance. A corollary, suggested by data from prospective studies (74), is that the more insulin resistant among a group of individuals of normal body weight will be protected from future weight gain. However, this is only a theory and is by no means universally accepted (75). In addition, insulin resistance is clearly maladaptive in terms of risk of CVD and other chronic diseases.

Insulin normally inhibits fat mobilization from adipose tissue and activates LPL. These are both metabolic processes that become insulin resistant in obesity. However, in contrast to the direct regulation of insulin secretion by plasma glucose concentration, the regulation of insulin secretion by fat metabolites is relatively weak. This means that oversecretion of insulin (due to insulin resistance) compensates for defects in glucose metabolism to a much greater degree than for defects in lipid metabolism. Disruption of the postprandial response by insulin leads to the dyslipidaemic state (section 4.8.2). Differential insulin resistance of specific organs or tissues may account for regional fat accumulation. For instance, the relative insulin sensitivity of intra-abdominal fat is thought to be required for central fat accumulation.

Physical activity improves insulin sensitivity through weight reduction and increased cardiorespiratory fitness. However, it also improves insulin sensitivity independently of these factors (76).

Hormones affecting reproductive function
Significant associations are seen in reproductive endocrinology between excess body fat, particularly abdominal obesity, and ovulatory dysfunction, hyperandrogenism and hormone-sensitive carcinomas (77). Changes in circulating sex hormones appear to underlie these abnormalities. Androstenedione and testosterone concentrations are commonly elevated whereas that of sex hormone binding globulin (SHBG) is reduced, while the plasma ratio of estrone to estradiol is also increased in obesity. A decrease in SHBG is associated with an increased clearance of free testosterone and estradiol, resulting in a disturbed sex hormone equilibrium.

Moderate obesity is frequently associated with polycystic ovary syndrome, which is the most common endocrine disorder of reproduction (78). Obesity contributes to or worsens, and weight loss generally improves, the associated hormonal abnormalities and menstrual function of obese women with polycystic ovary syndrome (79).

Adrenocortical function

Obese subjects have a normal circulating plasma cortisol concentration with a normal circadian rhythm, and normal urinary free cortisol. However, the cortisol production rate is increased in obesity to compensate for an accelerated rate of cortisol breakdown (*80, 81*). Cortisol inhibits the antilipolytic effect of insulin in human adipocytes, an effect that may normally be particularly pronounced in abdominal fat because it contains a high density of glucocorticoid receptors. This mechanism may contribute to the manifestations of insulin resistance (*82*).

Studies have shown that patients with intra-abdominal fat accumulation have increased cortisol secretion, probably because they have increased activity of the hypothalamic–pituitary axis (HPA). Stress, alcohol and smoking have all been shown to stimulate the activity of the HPA (*83*).

4.8.2 *Metabolic disturbances*

Dyslipidaemia

Obese individuals are frequently characterized by a dyslipidaemic state in which plasma triglycerides are raised, HDL cholesterol concentrations are reduced and low-density lipoprotein apo B (LDL-apoB) levels are raised. This metabolic profile is most often seen in obese patients with a high accumulation of intra-abdominal fat and has consistently been related to an increased risk of CHD (*84*).

Excessive intra-abdominal fat accumulation is also associated with a greater proportion of small, dense low-density lipoprotein (LDL) particles. The high proportion of these small dense LDL particles may be the result of metabolic disturbances related to the accompanying high triglyceride or low HDL levels. Indeed, the hypertriglyceridaemic state may be the combined result of an increased production and a reduced breakdown of triglyceride-rich lipoproteins (*84, 85*). This process results in lower HDL cholesterol levels and favours the triglyceride enrichment of LDL. The triglyceride-rich LDL is then enzymically degraded by hepatic lipase to produce small, dense LDL particles. A large proportion of these particles cannot be identified simply by the measurement of total or LDL cholesterol levels because these cholesterol levels are frequently in the normal range in obese individuals. A better indicator of small, dense LDL particle levels is an elevated ratio of LDL-apoB to LDL cholesterol.

Impaired fat tolerance (i.e. prolonged and/or exaggerated lipaemia following fat ingestion) is now also recognized as a component both of insulin resistance and of the atherogenic lipoprotein phenotype (*86*).

The metabolic syndrome and obesity

The common association of obesity with other CVD risk factors is well recognized. This clustering has been given several labels, including syndrome X and the insulin resistance syndrome, but the term metabolic syndrome is now favoured. There is no internationally agreed definition of the syndrome, but a suitable working definition would include two or more of the following:

— impaired glucose tolerance;
— elevated blood pressure;
— hypertriglyceridaemia and low HDL cholesterol;
— insulin resistance;
— central obesity.

Insulin resistance and/or hyperinsulinaemia have been suggested as the underlying cause(s) linking these conditions (*87*). Each individual component of the syndrome increases the CVD risk but, in combination, they interact to increase risk in a synergistic fashion.

Epidemiological studies confirm that the metabolic syndrome occurs commonly in a wide variety of ethnic groups including Caucasoids, Afro-Americans, Mexican Americans, Asian Indians and Chinese, Australian Aborigines, Polynesians and Micronesians. However, there is some evidence that the patterns of risk factors observed vary between and even within populations (*88*).

4.9 Debilitating health problems associated with obesity

Before chronic, life-threatening illness develops, overweight and obese patients usually present to primary care physicians with a range of conditions that adversely affect their quality of life, are often mechanical in origin, and are caused by the large amounts of excess weight that have to be carried. Though often perceived as less serious, these conditions are nonetheless debilitating and sometimes painful; they may also be costly in terms of the health resources consumed in their treatment and the absences from work that they cause. Sleep apnoea can have fatal consequences associated with cardiac arrhythmias. Unfortunately, few data are available on the economic costs of these conditions attributable to obesity.

4.9.1 *Osteoarthritis and gout*

Obesity is associated with the development of osteoarthritis and gout and, in obese middle-aged women at or after menopause, pain at the medial aspect of the knee (adiposa dolorosa juxta-articularis). Possible factors underlying the relationship between obesity and osteo-arthritis include mechanical stresses related to the increased load carried by the obese, metabolic changes associated with increased fatness, and dietary elements (e.g. high fat content) related to the development of obesity. The data indicate that mechanical damage is usually the cause. The increased risk of gout associated with obesity may be related to the accompanying hyperuricaemia, although central fat distribution may also be involved, particularly in women (*89–91*).

4.9.2 *Pulmonary diseases*

Obesity impairs respiratory function and structure, leading to physiological and pathophysiological impairments. The work of breathing is increased in obesity, mainly as a result of the extreme stiffness of the thoracic cage consequent on the accumulation of adipose tissue in and around the ribs, abdomen and diaphragm (*92*). Hypoxaemia is common, partly because the low relaxation volume causes ventilation to occur at volumes below the closing volume (*93, 94*), and is exacerbated when lying down because of the reduced functional residual capacity (*95*).

Sleep apnoea occurs in more than 10% of men and women with a BMI of 30 or above, and 65–75% of individuals with obstructive sleep apnoea are obese. In one study, sleep apnoea occurred in 77% of those with a BMI above 40. In addition to BMI, however, obstructive sleep apnoea is related to central obesity and to neck size, probably as a result of the narrowing of the upper airway when lying down. The nocturnal disruption of sleep is associated with daytime somnolence, hypercapnia, morning headaches, pulmonary hypertension and, eventually, right ventricular failure (*96, 97*).

4.10 Psychological problems associated with obesity

The SOS study found that the proportion of individuals receiving pensions for medical reasons was more than twice as high in obese patients as in population controls. Psychological problems in the obese (with women more affected than men) were found to be worst in those who were also chronically ill or injured, e.g. suffering from rheumatoid arthritis, cancer or spinal injury (*98*). The true social and economic costs of the non-fatal health consequences of obesity may therefore be seriously underestimated.

Other data on the psychosocial aspects of obesity relate mainly to the USA, and reflect cultural differences that may be irrelevant to other countries, especially as there appear to be ethnic differences in attitudes towards obesity. Black women in the USA, for instance, are 2–3 times more likely than white women to be obese, yet black women have been shown to experience less social pressure to reduce their weight, start dieting later in life, and be significantly less likely to diet at each developmental milestone (*99*). Nevertheless, as the prevalence of obesity rises in developing countries, and populations are increasingly affected by the cultural values prevailing in industrialized countries, psychosocial problems are likely to become an increasingly common feature of the overall health profile of the obese.

It is important to note that the mechanisms leading to impaired psychological health are different from those underlying physical illness. The psychosocial problems associated with obesity are not the inevitable consequences of obesity but rather of the culture-bound values by which people view body fat as "unhealthy" and "ugly". Stunkard & Sobal (*100*) noted that ". . . obesity does not create a psychological burden. Obesity is a physical state. People create the psychological burden."

4.10.1 *Social bias, prejudice and discrimination*

Obesity is highly stigmatized in many industrialized countries, in terms both of the perceived undesirable bodily appearance and of the character defects that it is supposed to indicate. Even children as young as 6 years of age describe the silhouette of an obese child as "lazy", "dirty", "stupid", "ugly", "liar" and "cheat" more often than drawings of other body shapes (*101*).

Obese people have to contend with discrimination. Analyses of large surveys have shown that, compared with their non-obese peers, those who are obese are likely to complete fewer years at school, and less likely to be accepted by prestigious schools or to enter desirable professions. Furthermore, overweight young women in the United Kingdom and the USA earn significantly less than healthy women who are not overweight or than women with other chronic health problems (*102*).

The negative stereotypes and attitudes of health professionals (including doctors, medical students, nutritionists and nurses) towards obesity are of particular importance. Awareness of these negative attitudes may make the obese reluctant to seek medical assistance for their condition (*103*). Doctors may be less interested in managing overweight patients, believing that they are weak-willed and less likely to benefit from counselling. British general practitioners were less likely to prescribe lipid-lowering agents to overweight people (or to smokers), and doctors explicitly stated that this was their policy (*104*). Although little has been done so far to improve the stereotypes and attitudes of health professionals, Wiese et al. (*105*) found that educational intervention was associated with a more positive attitude to the obese among first-year medical students.

4.10.2 *Psychological effects*

Research in this area has produced inconclusive results. Scores on standard psychological tests have been shown to differ little, if at all, between obese and non-obese people, and the evaluation of self-esteem in obese children and adolescents has not given consistent results (*106*). However, the implication that obesity has no psychological consequences is in conflict with the experience of overweight individuals and with the literature, in which strong cultural bias and negative attitudes towards obese people are consistently reported. Friedman & Brownell (*107*) suggest that this "paradox" can be explained by the manner in which these first-generation studies have been conducted and that new studies should be carried out to examine risk factors within the obese population.

4.10.3 *Body shape dissatisfaction*

Many obese people have an altered body image, i.e. they see their bodies as ugly and believe that others wish to exclude them from social interaction. This occurs most often in young women of middle and upper socioeconomic status, among whom obesity is less prevalent, and in those who have been obese since childhood.

4.10.4 *Eating disorders*

Binge-eating disorder is a recognized psychological condition (*108*) that occurs with increased frequency among obese persons, approximately 30% of whom seek medical help in dealing with it. In particular, the disorder is associated with severe obesity, a high frequency of weight cycling, and pronounced psychiatric comorbidity. It is characterized mainly by uncontrolled binge-eating episodes, usually in the early evening or at night.

Obese binge-eaters have worse moods and more severe psychological problems than obese people who do not binge-eat, and are more likely to drop out of weight-control programmes based on behaviour modification. Although binge-eaters may regain weight faster than non-binge-eaters, both short- and long-term weight loss among binge-eaters and non-binge-eaters appears to be similar (*109*).

The night-eating syndrome is characterized by the consumption of at least 25% — although more recent opinion suggests up to 50% — of total energy intake after the evening meal. This syndrome seems to be more common in morbidly obese patients and is related to sleep disturbances such as sleep apnoea. It is thought to be due to alterations in the circadian rhythm, affecting both food intake and mood.

Nocturnal sleep-related disorder is a newly delineated night-eating pattern characterized by eating on arousal from sleep. It may be a variant of binge-eating disorder but its relationship with night-eating syndrome is unclear.

There is no clear evidence that these eating disorders are the primary cause of weight gain. It has been suggested that the increasing incidence of eating disorders is associated with the psychological pressure to slim (*110, 111*). The fact that these disorders do not exist in societies where obesity is accepted as normal strongly supports the view that they have a cultural basis. Once established in patients, however, they are serious medical conditions and are difficult to cure.

4.11 Health consequences of overweight and obesity in childhood and adolescence

4.11.1 *Prevalence*

Obesity-related symptoms in children and adolescents include psychosocial problems, increased CVD risk factors, abnormal glucose metabolism, hepatic–gastrointestinal disturbances, sleep apnoea and orthopaedic complications (Table 4.4).

The most important long-term consequence of childhood obesity is its persistence into adulthood, with all the associated health risks. Obesity is more likely to persist when its onset is in late childhood or adolescence and when the obesity is severe (*112, 113*). Overweight in adolescence has also been shown to be significantly associated with long-term mortality and morbidity (*114*).

Table 4.4
Health consequences of childhood obesity

High prevalence	Intermediate prevalence	Low prevalence
Faster growth	Hepatic steatosis	Orthopaedic complications
Psychosocial problems	Abnormal glucose metabolism	Sleep apnoea
Persistence into adulthood (for late-onset and severe obesity)	Persistence into adulthood (depending on age of onset and severity)	Polycystic ovary syndrome
		Pseudotumour cerebri
		Cholelithiasis
Dyslipidaemia		Hypertension

4.11.2 *Psychosocial effects*

The most common consequence of obesity in children in industrialized countries is poor psychosocial functioning. Preadolescent children associate the shape (or silhouette) of an overweight body with poor social functioning, impaired academic success and reduced fitness and health (*115*), as well as with character defects (see p. 56). However, there is little evidence to suggest that self-esteem is significantly affected in obese young children (*106, 116*).

Among teenagers, however, cross-sectional studies consistently show an inverse relationship between body weight and both overall self-esteem and body image (*106*). A marked self-awareness of body shape and physical appearance develops during adolescence so that it is perhaps not surprising that the pervasive, negative social messages associated with obesity in many communities have a major impact at this stage. Overweight in adolescence may also be associated with later social and economic problems. A large prospective study conducted in the USA has shown that women who were overweight during adolescence and young adulthood were more likely to have lower family incomes, higher rates of poverty and lower rates of marriage than women with various other forms of chronic physical disability during adolescence (*102*).

4.11.3 *Cardiovascular risk factors*

Dyslipidaemia, hypertension and insulin resistance are frequently seen in obese children (*117, 118*) and dyslipidaemia appears to be related to increased abdominal fat accumulation (*119*). Caprio and coworkers (*120*) suggest that insulin resistance in children may also be associated with abdominal obesity.

Although NIDDM is very rare, it accounts for one-third of all new cases of diabetes seen in some institutions in the USA (*121*).

Elevated serum lipid and lipoprotein levels, blood pressure and plasma insulin in childhood are all carried over into young adulthood, obesity status in childhood at baseline being a significant predictor of adult values (*122, 123*).

4.11.4 *Hepatic and gastric complications*

Hepatic complications in obese children have been reported, particularly hepatic steatosis characterized by raised serum transaminase levels (*124*). Abnormal liver enzymes may be associated with cholelithiasis, but this condition is rare in children and adolescents.

Gastro-oesophageal reflux and gastric emptying disturbances, which affect a minority of obese children, may be a consequence of raised intra-abdominal pressure due to increased abdominal fat.

4.11.5 *Orthopaedic complications*

It is well documented that obese children can suffer from orthopaedic complications. The more serious of these include slipped capital femoral epiphysis (*125*) and Blount disease (a bone deformity resulting from overgrowth of the tibia) (*126, 127*), while more minor abnormalities include knock knee (genu valgum) and increased susceptibility to ankle sprains.

4.11.6 *Other complications of childhood obesity*

Other serious complications to have been reported in obese children include obstructive sleep apnoea and pseudomotor cerebri. Obstructive sleep apnoea can cause hypoventilation and even sudden death in severe cases (*128, 129*). Pseudomotor cerebri is a rare condition linked to raised intracranial pressure; it requires immediate medical attention.

References

1. **Berrios X et al.** On behalf of the Inter-Health sites. Distribution and prevalence of major risk factors of noncommunicable diseases in selected countries: the WHO Inter-Health Programme. *Bulletin of the World Health Organization*, 1997, **75**:99–108.

2. **Bray G.** Coherent, preventive and management strategies for obesity. In: Chadwick DJ, Cardew GC, eds. *The origins and consequences of obesity*. Chichester, Wiley, 1996:228–254 (Ciba Foundation Symposium 201).

3. **Stamler J, Wentworth DN, Neaton JD.** Is relationship between serum cholesterol and risk of premature death from coronary heart disease continuous and graded? Findings in 356,222 primary screenees of the Multiple Risk Factor Intervention Trial (MRFIT). *Journal of the American Medical Association*, 1986, **256**:2823–2828.

4. **Stamler J, Neaton JD, Wentworth DN.** Blood pressure (systolic and diastolic) and risk of fatal coronary heart disease. *Hypertension*, 1989, 13(5 Suppl.):I2–I12.

5. **Manson JE, Willett WC, Stampfer MJ.** Body weight and mortality among women. *New England Journal of Medicine*, 1995, **333**:677–685.

6. **Kumanyika SK.** Special issues regarding obesity in minority populations. *Annals of Internal Medicine*, 1993, **119**:650–654.

7. **Fujimoto WY et al.** Susceptibility to development of central adiposity among populations. *Obesity Research*, 1995, **3**(Suppl. 2):179S–186S.

8. **Rebuffe-Strive M, Björntorp P.** Regional adipose tissue metabolism in man. In: Vague J, Björntorp P, Guy-Grand B, eds. *Metabolic complications of human obesities*. Amsterdam, Excerpta Medica, 1985:149–159.

9. **Manson JE et al.** Body weight and longevity: a reassessment. *Journal of the American Medical Association*, 1987, **257**:353–358.

10. **Seidell JC et al.** Overweight, underweight, and mortality. A prospective study of 48,287 men and women. *Archives of Internal Medicine*, 1996, **156**:958–963.

11. **Chan JM et al.** Obesity, fat distribution, and weight gain as risk factors for clinical diabetes in men. *Diabetes Care*, 1994, **17**:961–969.

12. **Rissanen A et al.** Risk of disability and mortality due to overweight in a Finnish population. *British Medical Journal*, 1990, **301**:835–837.

13. **Shaper AG.** Obesity and cardiovascular disease. In: Chadwick DJ, Cardew GC, eds. *The origins and consequences of obesity.* Chichester, Wiley, 1996:90–107 (Ciba Foundation Symposium 201).

14. **Lindsted K, Tonstad S, Kuzma JW.** Body mass index and patterns of mortality among Seventh-day Adventist men. *International Journal of Obesity*, 1991, **15**:397–406.

15. **Blackburn GL et al.** Report of the American Institute of Nutrition (AIN) Steering Committee on healthy weight. *Journal of Nutrition*, 1994, **124**:2240–2243.

16. **Gordon T, Doyle JT.** Weight and mortality in men: the Albany Study. *International Journal of Epidemiology*, 1988, **17**:77–81.

17. **Sidney S, Friedman GD, Siegelaub AB.** Thinness and mortality. *American Journal of Public Health*, 1987, **77**:317–322.

18. **Willett WC et al.** New weight guidelines for Americans: justified or injudicious. *American Journal of Clinical Nutrition*, 1991, **53**:1102–1103.

19. **Hubert HB et al.** Obesity as an independent risk factor for cardiovascular disease: a 26-year follow-up of participants in the Framingham Heart Study. *Circulation*, 1983, **67**:968–977.

20. **Manson JE et al.** A prospective study of obesity and risk of coronary heart disease in women. *New England Journal of Medicine*, 1990, **322**:882–889.

21. **Jousilahti P et al.** Body weight, cardiovascular risk factors and coronary mortality. 15 year follow-up of middle-aged men and women in eastern Finland. *Circulation*, 1996, **93**:1372–1379.

22. **Kannel WB, D'Agostino RB, Cobb JL.** Effect of weight on cardiovascular disease. *American Journal of Clinical Nutrition*, 1996, **63**(Suppl. 4):419S–422S.

23. **Han TS et al.** Waist circumference action levels in the identification of cardiovascular risk factors: prevalence study in a random sample. *British Medical Journal*, 1995, **311**:1401–1405.

24. **Willett WC et al.** Weight, weight change, and coronary heart disease in women. Risk within the "normal" weight range. *Journal of the American Medical Association*, 1995, **273**:461–465.

25. **Enas EA, Mehta J.** Malignant coronary artery disease in young Asian Indians: thoughts on pathogenesis, prevention, and therapy. *Clinical Cardiology*, 1995, **18**:131–135.

26. **Stamler R et al.** Weight and blood pressure: Findings in hypertension screening of 1 million Americans. *Journal of the American Medical Association*, 1978, **240**:1607–1610.

27. **Van Itallie TB.** Health implications of overweight and obesity in the United States. *Annals of Internal Medicine*, 1985, **103**:983–988.

28. **Pi-Sunyer FX.** Health implications of obesity. *American Journal of Clinical Nutrition*, 1991, **53**(6 Suppl.):1595S–1603S.

29. **Burton BT et al.** Health implications of obesity: an NIH Consensus Development Conference. *International Journal of Obesity*, 1985, **9**:155–170.

30. **MacMahon S et al.** Blood pressure, stroke and coronary heart disease. Part 1, prolonged differences in blood pressure: prospective observational studies corrected for the regression dilution bias. *Lancet*, 1990, **335**:765–774.

31. **Abbott RD et al.** Body mass index and thromboembolic stroke in nonsmoking men in older middle age. The Honolulu Heart Program. *Stroke*, 1994, **25**:2370–2376.

32. **Sjöström L.** Swedish Obese Subjects, SOS. An intervention study of obesity. In: Ailhaud G et al., eds. *Obesity in Europe 91*. London, John Libbey, 1992:299–306.

33. **Larsson B et al.** Abdominal adipose tissue distribution, obesity, and risk of cardiovascular disease and death: 13 year follow up of participants in the study of men born in 1913. *British Medical Journal Clinical Research Edition*, 1984, **288**:1401–1404.

34. **Lapidus L et al.** Distribution of adipose tissue and risk of cardiovascular disease and death: a 12 year follow up of participants in the population study of women in Gothenburg, Sweden. *British Medical Journal*, 1984, **289**:1257–1261.

35. **Brenner BM, Garcia DL, Anderson S.** Glomeruli and blood pressure. Less of one, more the other? *American Journal of Hypertension*, 1988, **1**:335–347.

36. **Pi-Sunyer FX.** Medical hazards of obesity. *Annals of Internal Medicine*, 1993, **119**:655–660.

37. **Schapira DV et al.** Visceral obesity and breast cancer risk. *Cancer*, 1994, **74**:632–639.

38. **Le Marchand L, Wilkens LR, Mi MP.** Obesity in youth and middle age and risk of colorectal cancer in men. *Cancer Causes and Control*, 1992, **3**:349–354.

39. **Wolk A, Lindblad P, Adami HO.** Nutrition and renal cell cancer. *Cancer Causes and Control*, 1996, **7**:5–18.

40. **Swanson CA et al.** Body size and breast cancer risk among women under age 45 years. *American Journal of Epidemiology*, 1996, **143**:698–706.

41. **Wing RR et al.** Weight gain at the time of menopause. *Archives of Internal Medicine*, 1991, **151**:97–102.

42. **Lew EA, Garfinkel L.** Variations in mortality by weight among 750,000 men and women. *Journal of Chronic Diseases*, 1979, **32**:563–576.

43. **Frisch RE et al.** Lower lifetime occurrence of breast cancer and cancers of the reproductive system among former college athletes. *American Journal of Clinical Nutrition*, 1987, **45**:328–335.

44. Albanes D, Blair A, Taylor PR. Physical activity and risk of cancer in the NHANES I population. *American Journal of Public Health*, 1989, **79**:744–750.

45. Hartz AJ et al. Relationship of obesity to diabetes: influence of obesity level and body fat distribution. *Preventive Medicine*, 1983, **12**:351–357.

46. Haffner SM et al. Do upper-body and centralized adiposity measure different aspects of regional body-fat distribution? Relationship to non-insulin-dependent diabetes mellitus, lipids, and lipoproteins. *Diabetes*, 1987, **36**:43–51.

47. van Noord PA et al. The relationship between fat distribution and some chronic diseases in 11,825 women participating in the DOM-project. *International Journal of Epidemiology*, 1990, **19**:546–570.

48. Dowse GK et al. Abdominal obesity and physical inactivity as risk factors for NIDDM and impaired glucose tolerance in Indian, Creole, and Chinese Mauritians. *Diabetes Care*, 1991, **14**:271–282.

49. Shelgikar KM, Hockaday TD, Yajnik CS. Central rather than generalized obesity is related to hyperglycaemia in Asian Indian subjects. *Diabetic Medicine*, 1991, **8**:712–717.

50. Skarfors ET, Selinus KI, Lithell HO. Risk factors for developing non-insulin dependent diabetes: a 10 year follow-up of men in Uppsala. *British Medical Journal*, 1991, **303**:755–760.

51. McKeigue PM et al. Relationship of glucose intolerance and hyperinsulinaemia to body fat pattern in south Asians and Europeans. *Diabetologia*, 1992, **35**:785–791.

52. Schmidt M et al. Associations of waist-hip ratio with diabetes mellitus. Strength and possible modifiers. *Diabetes Care*, 1992, **15**:912–914.

53. Tai TY et al. Association of body build with non-insulin-dependent diabetes mellitus and hypertension among Chinese adults: a 4-year follow-up study. *International Journal of Epidemiology*, 1992, **21**:511–517.

54. Marshall JA et al. Ethnic differences in risk factors associated with the prevalence of non-insulin-dependent diabetes mellitus. The San Luis Valley Diabetes Study. *American Journal of Epidemiology*, 1993, **137**:706–718.

55. Shaten BJ et al. Risk factors for the development of type II diabetes among men enrolled in the usual care group of the Multiple Risk Factor Intervention Trial. *Diabetes Care*, 1993, **16**:1331–1339.

56. Chou P, Liao MJ, Tsai ST. Associated risk factors of diabetes in Kin-Hu, Kinmen. *Diabetes Research and Clinical Practice*, 1994, **26**:229–235.

57. Collins VR et al. Increasing prevalence of NIDDM in the Pacific island population of Western Samoa over a 13-year period. *Diabetes Care*, 1994, **17**:288–296.

58. Ohlson LO et al. The influence of body fat distribution on the incidence of diabetes mellitus. 13.5 years of follow-up of the participants in the study of men born in 1913. *Diabetes*, 1985, **34**:1055–1058.

59. Modan M et al. Effect of past and concurrent body mass index on prevalence of glucose intolerance and type 2 (non-insulin-dependent) diabetes and on insulin response. *Diabetologia*, 1986, **29**:82–89.

60. **Lundgren H et al.** Adiposity and adipose tissue distribution in relation to incidence of diabetes in women: Results from a prospective population study in Gothenburg, Sweden. *International Journal of Obesity*, 1989, 13:413–423.

61. **Colditz GA et al.** Weight as a risk factor for clinical diabetes in women. *American Journal of Epidemiology*, 1990, **132**:501–513.

62. **Haffner SM et al.** Incidence of type II diabetes in Mexican Americans predicted by fasting insulin and glucose levels, obesity, and body-fat distribution. *Diabetes*, 1990, **39**:283–288.

63. **Charles MA et al.** Risk factors for NIDDM in white population. Paris prospective study. *Diabetes*, 1991, **40**:796–799.

64. **Knowler WC et al.** Obesity in the Pima Indians: its magnitude and relationship with diabetes. *American Journal of Clinical Nutrition*, 1991, 53(6 Suppl.):1543S–1551S.

65. **Cassano PA et al.** Obesity and body fat distribution in relation to the incidence of non-insulin-dependent diabetes mellitus. A prospective cohort study of men in the normative aging study. *American Journal of Epidemiology*, 1992, **136**:1474–1486.

66. **Chan JM et al.** Obesity, fat distribution, and weight gain as risk factors for clinical diabetes in men. *Diabetes Care*, 1994, 17:961–969.

67. **Schranz AG.** Abnormal glucose tolerance in the Maltese. A population-based longitudinal study of the natural history of NIDDM and IGT in Malta. *Diabetes Research and Clinical Practice*, 1989, 7:7–16.

68. **Helmrich SP et al.** Physical activity and reduced occurrence of non-insulin-dependent diabetes mellitus. *New England Journal of Medicine*, 1991, 325:147–152.

69. **O'Dea K.** Marked improvement in carbohydrate and lipid metabolism in diabetic Australian aborigines after temporary reversion to traditional lifestyle. *Diabetes*, 1984, **33**:596–603.

70. **Maclure KM et al.** Weight, diet, and the risk of symptomatic gallstones in middle-aged women. *New England Journal of Medicine*, 1989, **321**:563–569.

71. **Kissebah AH, Peiris AN.** Biology of regional body fat distribution. Relationship to non-insulin-dependent diabetes mellitus. *Diabetes/Metabolism Reviews*, 1989, 5:83–109.

72. **Seidell J et al.** Visceral fat accumulation in men is positively associated with insulin, glucose and C-peptide levels, but negatively with testosterone levels. *Metabolism: Clinical and Experimental*, 1990, 39:897–901.

73. **Eckel RH.** Insulin resistance: an adaptation for weight maintenance. *Lancet*, 1992, 340:1452–1453.

74. **Swinburn BA et al.** Insulin resistance associated with lower rates of weight gain in Pima Indians. *Journal of Clinical Investigation*, 1991, **88**:168–173.

75. **Wing RR.** Insulin sensitivity as a predictor of weight regain. *Obesity Research*, 1997, 5:24–29.

76. **Mikines KJ.** The influence of physical activity and inactivity on insulin action and secretion in man. *Acta Physiologica Scandinavica Supplement*, 1992, **609**:1–43.

77. **Kirschner MA et al.** Obesity, androgens, oestrogens, and cancer risk. *Cancer Research*, 1982, **42**(8 Suppl.):3281S–3285S.

78. **Dunaif A.** Polycystic ovary syndrome and obesity. In: Björntorp P, Brodoff BN, eds, *Obesity*. Philadelphia, Lippincott, 1992:594–605.

79. **Kiddy DS et al.** Improvement in endocrine and ovarian function during dietary treatment of obese women with polycystic ovary syndrome. *Clinical Endocrinology*, 1992, **36**:105–111.

80. **Migeon CJ, Green OC, Eckert JP.** Study of adrenocortical function in obesity. *Metabolism: Clinical and Experimental*, 1963, **12**:718–730.

81. **Galvão-Teles A et al.** Free cortisol in obesity: effect of fasting. *Acta Endocrinologica*, 1976, **81**:321–329.

82. **Cigolini M, Smith U.** Human adipose tissue in culture. VIII. Studies on the insulin-antagonistic effect of glucocorticoids. *Metabolism: Clinical and Experimental*, 1979, **28**:502–510.

83. **Björntorp P.** Endocrine abnormalities of obesity. *Metabolism: Clinical and Experimental*, 1995, **44**:21–23.

84. **Despres JP et al.** Regional distribution of body fat, plasma lipoproteins, and cardiovascular disease. *Arteriosclerosis*, 1990, **10**:497–511.

85. **Despres JP.** Obesity and lipid metabolism: relevance of body fat distribution. *Current Opinion in Lipidology*, 1991, **2**:5–15.

86. **Griffin BA, Zampelas A.** Influence of dietary fatty acids on the atherogenic lipoprotein phenotype. *Nutrition Research Reviews*, 1995, **8**:1–26.

87. **Ferrannini E et al.** Hyperinsulinaemia: the key feature of a cardiovascular and metabolic syndrome. *Diabetologia*, 1991, **34**:416–422.

88. **Hodge AM, Zimmet PZ.** The epidemiology of obesity. *Baillieres Clinical Endocrinology and Metabolism*, 1994, **8**:577–599.

89. **Davis MA et al.** Body fat distribution and osteoarthritis. *American Journal of Epidemiology*, 1990, **132**:701–707.

90. **Roubenoff R et al.** Incidence and risk factors for gout in white men. *Journal of the American Medical Association*, 1991, **266**:3004–3007.

91. **Felson DT et al.** Weight loss reduces the risk for symptomatic knee osteoarthritis in women. The Framingham Study. *Annals of Internal Medicine*, 1992, **116**:535–539.

92. **Naimark A, Cherniack RM.** Compliance of the respiratory system and its components in health and obesity. *Journal of Applied Physiology*, 1960, **15**:377–382.

93. **Holley HS et al.** Regional distribution of pulmonary ventilation and perfusion in obesity. *Journal of Clinical Investigation*, 1967, **46**:475–481.

94. **Don HF et al.** The measurement of gas trapped in the lungs at functional residual capacity and the effects of posture. *Anesthesiology*, 1971, **35**:582–590.

95. **Tucker DH, Sieker HO.** The effects of change in body position on lung volumes and intrapulmonary gas mixing in patients with obesity, heart failure and emphysema. *Journal of Clinical Investigation*, 1960, **39**:787–791.

96. **Vgontzas AN et al.** Sleep apnea and sleep disruption in obese patients. *Archives of Internal Medicine*, 1994, **154**:1705–1711.

97. **Strollo PJ Jr, Rogers RM.** Obstructive sleep apnea. *New England Journal of Medicine*, 1996, **334**:99–104.

98. **Sullivan M et al.** Swedish obese subjects (SOS) — an intervention study of obesity. Baseline evaluation of health and psychosocial functioning in the first 1743 subjects examined. *International Journal of Obesity and Related Metabolic Disorders*, 1993, **17**:503–512.

99. **Striegel-Moore RH et al.** Weight-related attitudes and behaviors of women who diet to lose weight: a comparison of black dieters and white dieters. *Obesity Research*, 1996, **4**:109–116.

100. **Stunkard AJ, Sobal J.** Psychological consequences of obesity. In: Brownell KD, Fairburn CG, eds. *Eating disorders and obesity: a comprehensive handbook*. London, Guilford Press, 1995:417–430.

101. **Staffieri JR.** A study of social stereotype of body image in children. *Journal of Personality and Social Psychology*, 1967, **7**:101–104.

102. **Gortmaker SL et al.** Social and economic consequences of overweight in adolescence and young adulthood. *New England Journal of Medicine*, 1993, **329**:1008–1012.

103. **De Jong W, Kreck RE.** The social psychological effects of overweight. In: Herman CP et al., eds. *Physical appearance, stigma and social behaviour. The Ontario Symposium, vol 3*. Hilsdale, Lawrence Erlbaum, 1986:66–87.

104. **Evans JS et al.** General practitioners' tacit and stated policies in the prescription of lipid-lowering agents. *British Journal of General Practice*, 1995, **45**:15–18.

105. **Wiese HJ et al.** Obesity stigma reduction in medical students. *International Journal of Obesity and Related Metabolic Disorders*, 1992, **16**:859–868.

106. **French SA, Story M, Perry CL.** Self-esteem and obesity in children and adolescents: a literature review. *Obesity Research*, 1995, **3**:479–490.

107. **Friedman M, Brownell KD.** Psychological correlates of obesity: moving to the next research generation. *Psychological Bulletin*, 1995, **117**:3–20.

108. *Diagnostic and statistical manual of mental disorders*, 4th ed. Washington, DC, American Psychiatric Association, 1994.

109. **Wing RR, Greeno CG.** Behavioural and psychosocial aspects of obesity and its treatment. *Baillieres Clinical Endocrinology and Metabolism*, 1994, **8**:689–703.

110. **Tiggemann M, Pickering AS.** Role of television in adolescent women's body dissatisfaction and drive for thinness. *International Journal of Eating Disorders*, 1996, **20**:199–203.

111. Nelson CL, Gidycz CA. A comparison of body image perception in bulimics, restrainers, and normal women: an extension of previous findings. *Addictive Behaviors*, 1993, **18**:503–509.

112. Abraham S, Collins G, Nordsieck M. Relationship of childhood weight status to morbidity in adults. *HSMHA Health Report*, 1971, **86**:273–284.

113. Guo SS et al. The predictive value of childhood body mass index values for overweight at age 35 years. *American Journal of Clinical Nutrition*, 1994, **59**:810–819.

114. Must A et al. Long-term morbidity and mortality of overweight adolescents. A follow-up of the Harvard Growth Study of 1922 to 1935. *New England Journal of Medicine*, 1992, **327**:1350–1355.

115. Hill AJ, Silver EK. Fat, friendless and unhealthy: 9-year old children's perception of body shape stereotypes. *International Journal of Obesity and Related Metabolic Disorders*, 1995, **19**:423–430.

116. Klesges RC et al. Relationship between psychosocial functioning and body fat in preschool children: a longitudinal investigation. *Journal of Consulting and Clinical Psychology*, 1992, **60**:793–796.

117. Lauer RM et al. Coronary heart disease risk factors in school children: The Muscatine study. *Journal of Pediatrics*, 1975, **86**:697–706.

118. Steinberger J et al. Relationship between insulin resistance and abnormal lipid profile in obese adolescents. *Journal of Pediatrics*, 1995, **126**:690–695.

119. Brambilla P et al. Peripheral and abdominal adiposity in childhood obesity. *International Journal of Obesity and Related Metabolic Disorders*, 1994, **18**:795–800.

120. Caprio S et al. Central adiposity and its metabolic correlates in obese adolescent girls. *American Journal of Physiology*, 1995, **269**:E118–E126.

121. Pinhas-Hamiel O et al. Increased incidence of non-insulin-dependent diabetes mellitus among adolescents. *Journal of Pediatrics*, 1996, **128**:608–615.

122. Bao W et al. Persistence of multiple cardiovascular risk clustering related to syndrome X from childhood to young adulthood. The Bogalusa Heart Study. *Archives of Internal Medicine*, 1994, **154**:1842–1847.

123. Raitakari OT et al. Clustering and six year cluster-tracking of serum total cholesterol, HDL-cholesterol and diastolic blood pressure in children and young adults. The Cardiovascular Risk in Young Finns Study. *Journal of Clinical Epidemiology*, 1994, **47**:1085–1093.

124. Noguchi H et al. The relationship between serum transaminase activities and fatty liver in children with simple obesity. *Acta Paediatrica Japonica*, 1995, **37**:621–625.

125. Loder RT. The demographics of slipped capital femoral epiphysis. An international multicenter study. *Clinical Orthopaedics and Related Research*, 1996, **322**:8–27.

126. Dietz WH Jr, Gross WL, Kirkpatrick JA Jr. Blount disease (tibia vara): another skeletal disorder associated with childhood obesity. *Journal of Pediatrics*, 1982, **101**:735–737.

127. **Henderson RC, Greene WB.** Etiology of late-onset tibia vara: is varus alignment a prerequisite? *Journal of Pediatric Orthopedics*, 1994, **14**:143–146.

128. **Silvestri JM et al.** Polysomnography in obese children with a history of sleep-associated breathing disorders. *Pediatric Pulmonology*, 1993, **16**:124–129.

129. **Riley DJ, Santiago TV, Edelman NH.** Complications of obesity-hypoventilation syndrome in childhood. *American Journal of Diseases in Children*, 1976, **130**:671–674.

5. Health benefits and risks of weight loss

5.1 Introduction

While the effects of obesity on the functioning, health, and quality of life of obese subjects have been studied in great detail, the impact of weight loss is less well documented. Short-term studies have demonstrated clear benefits from modest weight loss on most of the associated consequences of obesity but there are very few well designed studies on the benefits of long-term weight loss.

The health benefits and risks of weight loss and of maintaining the new lower weight in the long term are considered here with particular reference to mortality, general health, and obesity-related comorbidities including chronic diseases, endocrine and metabolic disturbances, and poor psychosocial functioning. Two distinct hazards of weight loss, namely gallstones and reduced bone density, are also considered, as is weight cycling. Finally, a brief account is given of the effects of weight loss in obese children and adolescents.

The following should be noted:

- Well designed studies of the effects of long-term (>2 years) weight loss are few in number. Difficulties associated with such studies include that of maintaining long-term weight loss, and the need to distinguish intentional from unintentional weight loss.

- Intentional weight loss results in marked improvements in NIDDM, dyslipidaemia, hypertension, cardiovascular risk and ovarian function. There are also improvements in breathlessness, sleep quality, sleep apnoea, back and joint pain, and osteoarthritis.

- The only distinct hazards of weight loss are an increased incidence of gallstones (when weight loss is rapid) and possibly a reduction in bone density.

5.2 Problems in evaluating the effects of long-term weight loss

Problems in evaluating the benefits of long-term weight loss include:

— the difficulty of maintaining weight loss in adults over a long period;
— whether weight cycling is taken into account, and how it is defined when the outcome of a study is assessed;
— distinguishing "unintentional" weight loss, which may reflect underlying disease, from "intentional" weight loss;
— distinguishing the beneficial effects of weight loss *per se* from those of the changes in diet and physical activity necessary to achieve it.

The distinction between intentional and unintentional weight loss is of major importance in studies of the relationships between weight loss and morbidity or mortality. If weight loss occurs unintentionally as a result of underlying disease or serious illness, the association between weight loss and morbidity or mortality will be artificially increased. A bias resulting from misclassification may also occur if only two weight measurements are made, especially if weight loss is temporary and due to a minor acute illness. For this reason it is recommended that a minimum of three — and preferably more — weight measurements should be made throughout the study period.

5.3 Weight loss and general health

5.3.1 Modest weight loss

Data from a number of studies have shown that modest weight loss (defined as a weight loss of up to 10%) improves glycaemic control, and reduces both blood pressure and cholesterol levels (1). Modest weight loss also improves lung function and breathlessness, reduces the frequency of sleep apnoea, improves sleep quality, and reduces daytime somnolence. However, the degree of improvement often depends on the length of time that the condition has been present. Modest weight loss will also alleviate osteoarthritis, depending on the degree of structural damage, as well as back and joint pain.

5.3.2 Extensive weight loss

Following vertical-banded gastroplasty, severely obese patients who lose 20–30 kg in weight, at a rate of 4.5 kg per month for the first 6 months, gain substantial health benefits. They show a marked fall in blood lipids within the first 2 years of follow-up, and the condition of 43% of hypertensive patients and 69% of NIDDM patients is improved. Furthermore, at the population level, the incidences of hypertension, hyperlipidaemia and NIDDM are reduced to about one-sixth of those seen in obese patients who maintain their excess weight (2, 3).

5.4 Weight loss and mortality

Unfortunately, most studies on weight loss and mortality have not controlled for unintentional weight loss or for cigarette smoking. In one large study of overweight white women in the USA in which these variables were evaluated, intentional weight loss consistently reduced mortality in women with obesity-related comorbidities such as NIDDM or CVD. However, the effects in women without comorbidities were not consistent with an association between intentional weight loss and reduction in mortality. Thus the benefit of intentional weight loss was best seen in those of poorer health status (*4*).

In a randomized controlled dietary intervention trial of post-infarct patients in India, the effect of dietary intervention on cardiac mortality was greatest among patients who had also lost around 10% of their body weight (*5*). Further longer-term, well controlled studies are thus clearly needed to define accurately the beneficial effects of weight loss on mortality.

5.5 Impact of weight loss on chronic disease, and on endocrine and metabolic disturbances

5.5.1 *Cardiovascular disease and hypertension*

A number of cardiovascular risk factors related to blood clotting (haemostatic, rheological and fibrinolytic) have been associated with overweight (*6–8*). In particular, coagulation factors VII and X, which are directly associated with BMI, are involved in thrombosis (*9*) and increased risk of myocardial infarction (*10*). Weight loss in overweight subjects has been shown to reduce red blood cell aggregation and to improve fibrinolytic capacity.

Weight loss induces a fall in blood pressure. Short trials lasting a few weeks show that each 1% reduction in body weight leads, on average, to a fall of 1 mmHg (0.133 kPa) systolic and 2 mmHg (0.267 kPa) diastolic pressure (*11–14*). Marked falls in blood pressure can occur with very-low-energy diets, although modest dietary restrictions are also beneficial. Antihypertensive drug therapy, reducing a high alcohol intake, and lowering both dietary salt intake (*15, 16*), and saturated fat intake (*17, 18*) all contribute to further blood-pressure reduction independently of weight loss. It is estimated that a 10-kg weight loss can produce a fall of 10 mmHg (1.33 kPa) in systolic blood pressure and of 20 mmHg (2.67 kPa) in diastolic pressure (*19*).

Longer trials, with a 10-year follow-up of patients identified originally as mildly hypertensive, show that positive dietary change, together with smoking cessation and an increase in isotonic exercise (e.g. running), reduces both body weight and blood pressure. These levels can be sustained for 10 years and the need for drug therapy is significantly reduced (*12*).

5.5.2 *Diabetes mellitus and insulin resistance*

Studies of weight loss in NIDDM patients have consistently shown that a weight reduction of 10–20% in obese individuals with NIDDM results in marked improvements in glycaemic control and insulin sensitivity. These improvements can last from 1 to 3 years even if the weight is subsequently regained. In the 75% of newly diagnosed NIDDM patients who are overweight, a 15–20% weight loss in the first year after diagnosis seems to reverse the elevated mortality risk of NIDDM (20). However, not all NIDDM patients respond to weight loss with metabolic improvements: the loss of abdominal adipose tissue may be more important in improvements in diabetic control than loss of weight per se.

Hyperglycaemia frequently decreases as soon as a low-energy diet is initiated, suggesting that dietary energy restriction has a beneficial effect independently of weight loss. Exercise training also improves glucose tolerance and insulin sensitivity independently of weight loss. The American Diabetes Association (21) recommends that aerobic exercise should be performed at moderate intensity for 20–45 minutes, 3 days per week. However, although epidemiological studies have emphasized the value of vigorous activity, mainly because it is easy to assess, total energy expenditure may be the important factor in limiting NIDDM rather than periods of intense physical activity (22).

5.5.3 Dyslipidaemia

The levels of blood lipids associated with obesity, namely high triacylglycerides, high cholesterol and low HDL cholesterol, can also be expected to return to normal after modest weight loss. For every 1 kg lost, LDL cholesterol has been estimated to decrease by 1% (23).

A 10-kg weight loss can produce a fall of 10% in total cholesterol levels, a 15% decrease in LDL levels, a 30% decrease in triacylglycerides and an 8% increase in HDL cholesterol (19). In addition, it has been found that serum triglyceride and HDL cholesterol levels show the most favourable changes after weight loss in those with a high waist:hip ratio (24).

5.5.4 Ovarian function

A weight loss of 5% or more during dietary treatment can improve insulin sensitivity and ovarian function in overweight and obese women with hirsutism and polycystic ovaries (25). In some obese women with amenorrhoea, normal menstrual function may be restored after weight loss (26).

5.6 Weight loss and psychosocial functioning

Most studies on the quality of life of obese patients before and after weight loss have been conducted on patients following surgery for obesity, and all show dramatic improvements in the overall quality of life. The SOS study in Sweden (27), for example, showed significant improvements in social interaction, anxiety, depression and mental well-being that were sustained for 2 years after surgery for obesity. Although it is unclear whether these improvements will be seen with modest weight loss following non-surgical intervention, Klem et al. (28) recently reported that formerly obese subjects who had lost weight through diet and/or exercise modification found their quality of life to be substantially improved. While this is based on self-reporting by individuals who were maintaining weight losses of at least 13.6 kg for periods of over 1 year, it provides additional evidence of the benefits of weight loss.

Dieting is often perceived to have untoward psychological effects, including depression, nervousness and irritability. However, studies have shown that weight loss is associated with a decrease in depression score, particularly when it is achieved by behaviour modification (29, 30).

A dramatic example of how extremely overweight individuals perceive their disorder has been provided by studies of a group of severely obese patients before and after losing weight as a result of gastric surgery (31, 32). Before surgery, all the patients felt unattractive and the great majority felt that people talked about them behind their backs at work. They also felt that they had been discriminated against when applying for jobs and treated disrespectfully by the medical profession. After having achieved a weight loss of 50 kg, all the patients said that they would prefer to be deaf, dyslexic or diabetic or to suffer from severe heart disease or acne than to return to their previous weight. Given a hypothetical choice, they all preferred to be of normal weight than have "a couple of million dollars" — a choice that they made in less than a second.

5.7 Hazards of weight loss

Weight loss from "crash" dieting may result in acute attacks of gout. However, for intentional and controlled weight loss resulting from medical intervention, only two distinct hazards have emerged from a variety of prospective studies:

- *Gallbladder disease.* Women who lose 4–10 kg have a 44% increased risk of clinically relevant gallstone disease, and greater weight loss increases this risk. Mobilization of cholesterol from adipose tissue stores is increased during weight loss, so that the risk of supersaturation of bile with cholesterol is greater than when weight is stable. Premenopausal women are at particular risk because of an estrogen-induced enhanced biliary secretion of cholesterol.

- *Reduced bone density*. Bone density is typically increased in obese patients and reduced after weight loss. In white women, weight loss beginning at age 50 was found to increase the risk of hip fracture (*33*). Whether there is restitution of bone mass with weight regain following slimming, however, is uncertain; Compston et al. (*34*) found this to be the case whereas Avenell et al. (*35*) did not. There is little information on the impact of weight cycling on bone density.

It should also be noted that, in societies in which overweight and obesity are seen as a sign of affluence, weight loss may be interpreted as an indication of financial disaster.

5.8 Weight cycling

Weight cycling refers to the repeated loss and regain of weight that can occur as a result of recurrent dieting. However, there is no standard definition of weight cycling so that comparison between different studies is difficult (*36*).

It has been suggested that weight cycling is associated with negative health outcomes, makes future weight loss more difficult and results in a decrease in lean-to-fat tissue ratio (*37*). However, the evidence is conflicting; weight variability was associated with increased risk of CVD and all-cause mortality in men, particularly in those who continued to smoke, but the association between weight change and death was not seen in the heaviest men (*38*). Recently in the USA, the National Task Force on the Prevention and Treatment of Obesity (*39*) concluded that the evidence available at the time was that the increased risk was not sufficient to outweigh the potential benefits of moderate weight loss in obese patients.

5.9 Effects of weight loss in obese children and adolescents

Weight loss of only 3% significantly decreased blood pressure in obese adolescents, and blood pressure was further improved if exercise was added to the weight-loss programme (*40*). A weight loss of nearly 16% in obese children resulted in a parallel decrease in serum triacylglycerides and plasma insulin in the first year, with an increase in HDL cholesterol. These changes remained stable in the second year of the study; after 5 years, body weight was still 13% below the initial value, peripheral hyperinsulinaemia was reduced and HDL cholesterol remained higher (*41*).

The symptoms of hepatic steatosis in obese children eventually disappear when excess weight is lost (*42*).

References

1. **Goldstein DJ.** Beneficial health effects of modest weight loss. *International Journal of Obesity*, 1992, **16**:397–415.

2. **Pories WJK et al.** Surgical treatment of obesity and its effect on diabetes: 10 year follow-up. *American Journal of Clinical Nutrition*, 1992, **55**(2 Suppl.):582S–585S.

3. **Sjöström L,** personal communication, 1995. Quoted in Bray GA, Coherent preventative and management strategies for obesity. In: Chadwick DJ, Cardew GC, eds. *The origins and consequences of obesity.* Chichester, Wiley, 1996:228–254 (Ciba Foundation Symposium 201).

4. **Williamson DF et al.** Prospective study of intentional weight loss and mortality in never-smoking overweight US white women aged 40–64 years. *American Journal of Epidemiology*, 1995, **141**:1128–1141.

5. **Singh RB et al.** Effect on mortality and reinfarction of adding fruits and vegetables to a prudent diet in the Indian experiment of infarct survival (IEIS). *Journal of the American College of Nutrition*, 1993, **12**:255–261.

6. **Ernst E, Matrai A.** Normalisation of hemorrheologic abnormalities during weight reduction in obese patients. *Nutrition*, 1987, **3**:337–339.

7. **Meade TW et al.** Fibrinolytic activity, clotting factors and long-term incidence of ischaemic heart disease in the Northwick Park Heart Study. *Lancet*, 1993, **342**:1076–1079.

8. Department of Health. *Nutritional aspects of cardiovascular disease. Report on health and social subjects 46.* London, Her Majesty's Stationery Office, 1994.

9. **Meade TW, Imeson J, Stirling Y.** Effects of changes in smoking and other characteristics on clotting factors and the risk of ischaemic heart disease. *Lancet*, 1987, ii:986–988.

10. **Böttiger LE, Carlson LA.** Risk factors for death for males and females. A study of the death pattern in the Stockholm prospective study. *Acta Medica Scandinavica*, 1982, **211**:437–442.

11. **Reisin E et al.** Effect of weight loss without salt restriction on the reduction in blood pressure in overweight hypertensive patients. *New England Journal of Medicine*, 1978, **298**:1–6.

12. **Stamler J et al.** Prevention and control of hypertension by nutritional–hygienic means. Long-term experience of the Chicago Coronary Prevention Evaluation Program. *Journal of the American Medical Association*, 1980, **243**:1819–1823.

13. **Tuck ML et al.** The effect of weight reduction on blood pressure, plasma renin activity and plasma aldosterone levels in obese patients. *New England Journal of Medicine*, 1981, **304**:930–933.

14. **Rissanen A et al.** Treatment of hypertension in obese patients; efficacy and feasibility of weight and salt reduction programs. *Acta Medica Scandinavica*, 1985, **218**:149–156.

15. Law MR, Frost CD, Wald NJ. By how much does dietary salt reduction lower blood pressure? III — Analysis of data from trials of salt reduction. *British Medical Journal*, 1991, **302**:819–824.

16. Elliott P et al. Intersalt revisited: further analyses of 24 hour sodium excretion and blood pressure within and across populations. *British Medical Journal*, 1996, **312**:1249–1253.

17. Ferro-Luzzi A et al. Changing the Mediterranean diet: effects on blood lipids. *American Journal of Clinical Nutrition*, 1984, **40**:1027–1037.

18. Puska P et al. Dietary fat and blood pressure: an intervention study on the effects of a low-fat diet with two levels of polyunsaturated fat. *Preventive Medicine*, 1985, **14**:573–584.

19. *Obesity in Scotland. Integrating prevention with weight management. A national clinical guideline recommended for use in Scotland.* Edinburgh, Scottish Intercollegiate Guidelines Network, 1996.

20. Lean MEJ et al. Obesity, weight loss and prognosis in type 2 diabetes. *Diabetic Medicine*, 1990, **7**:228–233.

21. American Diabetes Association Position Statement. Diabetes mellitus and exercise. *Diabetes Care*, 1995, **7**:416–420.

22. Wareham NJ et al. Glucose tolerance has a continuous relationship with total energy expenditure. *Diabetologia*, 1996, **39**(Suppl. 1):A8.

23. Dattilo AM, Kris-Etherton PM. Effects of weight reduction on blood lipids and lipoproteins: a meta-analysis. *American Journal of Clinical Nutrition*, 1992, **56**:320–328.

24. Hankey CR et al. Weight loss improves established indices of ischaemic heart disease risk. *Proceedings of the Nutrition Society*, 1995, **54**(Pt 2):94A.

25. Kiddy DS et al. Improvement in endocrine and ovarian function during dietary treatment of obese women with polycystic ovary syndrome. *Clinical Endocrinology*, 1992, **36**:105–111.

26. Pasquali R et al. Clinical and hormonal characteristics of obese amenhorrheic hyperandrogenic women before and after weight loss. *Journal of Clinical Endocrinology and Metabolism*, 1989, **68**:173–179.

27. Sjöström L, Narbro K, Sjöström D. Costs and benefits when treating obesity. *International Journal of Obesity and Related Metabolic Disorders*, 1995, **19**(Suppl. 6):S9–S12.

28. Klem ML et al. A descriptive study of individuals successful at long-term weight maintenance of substantial weight loss. *American Journal of Clinical Nutrition*, 1997, **66**:239–246.

29. Smoller JW, Wadden TA, Stunkard AJ. Dieting and depression: a critical review. *Journal of Psychosomatic Research*, 1987, **31**:429–440.

30. Kunesova M et al. Predictors of the weight loss in morbidly obese women: one year follow up. *International Journal of Obesity and Related Metabolic Disorders*, 1996, **20**(Suppl. 4):59.

31. Rand CSW, MacGregor AMC. Morbidly obese patients' perceptions of social discrimination before and after surgery for obesity. *Southern Medical Journal*, 1990, **83**:1390–1395.

32. **Rand CSW, MacGregor AMC.** Successful weight loss following obesity surgery and the perceived liability of morbid obesity. *International Journal of Obesity*, 1991, **15**:577–579.

33. **Langlois JA et al.** Weight change between age 50 years and old age is associated with risk of hip fracture in white women aged 67 years and older. *Archives of Internal Medicine*, 1996, **156**:989–994.

34. **Compston JE et al.** Effect of diet-induced weight loss on total body bone mass. *Clinical Science*, 1992, **82**:429–432.

35. **Avenell A et al.** Bone loss associated with a high fibre weight reduction diet in postmenopausal women. *European Journal of Clinical Nutrition*, 1994, **48**:561–566.

36. **Jeffery RW.** Does weight cycling present a health risk? *American Journal of Clinical Nutrition*, 1996, **63**(3 Suppl.):452S–455S.

37. **Lissner L et al.** Body weight variability in men: metabolic rate, health and longevity. *International Journal of Obesity*, 1990, **14**:373–383.

38. **Blair SN et al.** Body weight change, all-cause mortality and cause-specific mortality in the Multiple Risk Factor Intervention Trial. *Annals of Internal Medicine*, 1993, **119**:749–757.

39. Weight cycling. National Task Force on the Prevention and Treatment of Obesity. *Journal of the American Medical Association*, 1994, **272**:1196–1202.

40. **Rocchini AP et al.** Blood pressure in obese adolescents: effect of weight loss. *Pediatrics*, 1988, **82**:16–23.

41. **Knip M, Nuutinen O.** Long-term effects of weight reduction on serum lipids and plasma insulin in obese children. *American Journal of Clinical Nutrition*, 1993, **57**:490–493.

42. **Vajro P et al.** Persistent hyperaminotransferasemia resolving after weight loss in obese children. *Journal of Pediatrics*, 1994, **125**:239–241.

6. Economic costs of overweight and obesity

6.1 Introduction

The economic costs of overweight and obesity are important issues for health care providers and policy-makers alike. To date, there have been only a few attempts to quantify the economic burden of obesity-related morbidity and mortality. This is in marked contrast to smoking and alcohol consumption, where a large number of international studies have been undertaken to determine the magnitude of the economic burden that they impose on the community. In addition, few studies have assessed the relative cost-effectiveness of alternative interventions aimed at either preventing or treating obesity.

The limited information available on the economics of overweight and obesity is reviewed in this section. The use and limitations of cost-of-illness studies on obesity-related disease are summarized and the basic steps required in undertaking such a study are then outlined. A brief overview of the few studies in different countries that have provided estimates of the economic costs of obesity follows; key findings as well as the limitations of the methods used are highlighted, after which the cost-effectiveness of alternative interventions aimed at either preventing or treating obesity is reviewed. Finally, the implications of current understanding of the economics of obesity for public policy decision-making are considered and priorities for future research in this area discussed.

The following important points should be noted:

- The economic cost is made up of three main components:
  - "direct costs", i.e. the costs, to the individual and the service provider, associated with treating obesity itself;
  - the "opportunity cost" to the individual, i.e. the social and personal loss associated with obesity, generally arising from premature death or attributable morbidity;
  - "indirect costs", usually measured as lost production due to absenteeism from work and to premature death.
- The economic impact of obesity-related disease is usually estimated from cost-of-illness studies. These are useful in the development of public health policy but their limitations should be recognized: intangible costs and many of the direct costs of disease management and prevention, especially those incurred outside the formal health care system, tend to be ignored. A number of studies have therefore focused on the impact of obesity on broader social and economic issues, including the frequency of long-term sick leave.

- The economic costs of obesity have been assessed in several developed countries and are in the range 2–7% of total health care costs. These are conservative estimates based on variable criteria but clearly indicate that obesity represents one of the largest items of expenditure in national health care budgets.
- Although there have been no studies of the economic impact of obesity in developing countries, the escalating economic burden of adult NCDs in such countries has already been recognized by a number of international agencies including WHO and the World Bank. The real costs of therapy in developing countries exceed those in developed countries because of the extra burden associated with the use of scarce foreign exchange to pay for imports of expensive equipment and drugs, as well as the need for the specialized training of staff. In view of the existing burdens of endemic deficiency disorders and infectious diseases, obesity prevention is not only crucial but also the only sensible approach to planning public health policies in developing countries.
- Preliminary data suggest that a large proportion of the economic costs of obesity can be avoided by efficient prevention or intervention strategies.

6.2 Cost-of-illness studies

"Cost-of-illness" or "disease-costing" is a technique used to estimate the financial impact of disease on a community. The economic costs of obesity include:

- *Direct costs*: the cost to the *community* resulting from the diversion of resources to the diagnosis and treatment of diseases directly related to obesity, as well as from the cost of obesity treatment itself (including the cost of providing health care services to patients and their families, and the cost of service providers).

- *Intangible costs*: the cost to the *individual* arising from the impact of obesity on quality of life generally and on health specifically.

- *Indirect costs*: the welfare and economic benefits lost to *other members of society* through a reduction in the goods and services produced i.e. the impact of the reduced quality of life of the obese individual on the productive potential available to the rest of society. These costs are usually measured as the production lost through work-related absenteeism and premature death.

Most cost-of-illness studies focus on measuring direct and indirect costs, while less attention is given to the more difficult task of quantifying the intangible costs.

6.2.1 *Uses of cost-of-illness studies*

Cost-of-illness studies are useful in the development of public policy because they can:

- Identify and analyse how resources are currently being allocated to different types of costs, services and diseases.

- Help to identify potential improvements in health status, in the case of a specific disease, that can be achieved by the application of effective prevention programmes, or to identify a risk factor for a disease. A knowledge of the incidence and prevalence of the disease, the consequent use of health services, and costs can allow a calculation of the potential savings to a community that can be achieved through effective prevention programmes, which may (or may not) be greater than the costs of prevention.

- Assist health planners to make comparisons between the relative economic burden of different diseases that may assist in setting priorities for prevention, if taken together with information on the costs and effectiveness of prevention strategies.

- Provide data on the cost side of the cost–effectiveness ratio for subsequent economic appraisal.

- Be used to demonstrate to policy-makers and politicians the magnitude of the health problem in financial terms.

6.2.2 *Limitations of cost-of-illness studies*

The major criticism of cost-of-illness studies is that they can be misused. A cost-of-illness study may indicate that a disease is costly to treat. It may also suggest that a disease has a high social cost relative to other diseases or social problems, implying that society would be relatively better off without it. While this is obviously true, it does not mean that a higher priority should be given to treating that disease. Treatment (or prevention) may be relatively ineffective or expensive, so that priority-setting should be based on the relative cost-effectiveness of interventions and not on the cost of the disease alone. This criticism is best explained by Davey & Leeder (*1*):

> "... *Instead of answering the question, 'Where should I put the next health care dollar to achieve the greatest health gain?' cost-of-illness studies provide information only about the burden of illness. They concentrate on cost and say nothing about the effectiveness of treatment and value for money invested.*"

Some economists have argued that, while cost-of-illness studies do not indicate where resources should be allocated in the short term, they do indicate where the greatest potential health improvements and savings in health care resources could be made if effective interventions were available.

A further criticism concerns the focus of cost-of-illness studies on direct health care costs and the indirect costs of lost production, less emphasis being placed on the burden of disease, premature death and reduced quality of life. Because these latter intangible costs are less easy to measure in monetary terms, they tend to be ignored. Diseases associated with high health care costs but relatively low morbidity and mortality (such as dental disease) may therefore be seen as imposing a far greater burden than other diseases associated with high costs in terms of premature death and reduction in quality of life but low health care costs (such as youth suicide).

The definition of health care incorporated in cost-of-illness studies tends to be narrow and ignores many of the direct costs of disease management and prevention, especially those arising outside the formal health care system. This is particularly true of obesity, as the highest direct cost category is most likely to be the personal expenditure on weight-loss programmes incurred by overweight and obese individuals. The impact of the narrow range of direct costs included in studies is likely to vary across disease types and risk factors.

6.2.3 *Steps in undertaking a cost-of-illness study*

The following basic steps need to be taken in carrying out a cost-of-illness study on obesity-related disease where, in accordance with the WHO criteria, overweight is defined as BMI 25–29.9 and obesity as BMI $\geq$ 30:

— identify those diseases related to overweight and obesity;
— quantify the relationship between obesity and the associated disease morbidity and mortality using standard criteria (i.e. the population-attributable fractions (PAFs); for more information on PAFs, see below);
— identify the relevant economic cost categories to be estimated;
— quantify the total costs associated with diet-related disease;
— use the PAFs to apportion that share of total costs directly attributable to overweight and obesity;
— undertake a sensitivity analysis of key epidemiological and economic parameters (or assumptions) to provide a range of cost estimates.

Population-attributable fraction
The epidemiological statistic needed to quantify the direct relationship between a risk factor of interest and a disease (and thus quantify its associated economic costs) is the population-attributable fraction.

This has been defined as the proportion of total events (e.g. deaths or morbidity) in a population that could be prevented if a particular risk factor (e.g. obesity) could be eliminated.

The PAF reflects the overall impact of the morbidity and mortality associated with a factor (e.g. obesity) in the specified population. It can be interpreted from an etiological standpoint (causal outcomes attributed to a particular risk factor) or from a prevention standpoint (the maximum number of events that could be prevented). Many epidemiologists use the concept of "preventable proportion" as a useful generalization of the PAF concept.

Where only one category of exposure (e.g. obese or non-obese) is concerned, PAF is given by:

$$PAF = \frac{p(RR-1)}{1 + p(RR-1)}$$

where p = prevalence of risk factor (e.g. obesity) in a population
RR = relative risk
= incidence of disease in an obese person (I_e) divided by the incidence of disease in a non-obese person (I_o) = I_e/I_o

PAF can be expressed either as a fraction or as a percentage. Thus a PAF of 0.73 means that 73% of the incidence of the disease could be eliminated by removal of the risk factor (or conversely, that the risk factor is responsible for 73% of the incidence of the disease).

A number of epidemiological studies have assessed the relative risk of specific diseases associated with excess body weight. Most have used BMI as the risk factor; in only a few studies has the risk of disease been quantified in terms of body fat distribution (e.g. by the use of the waist circumference). Such studies have shown a positive relationship between BMI and the development of CHD (2–4), hypertension (5), stroke (6), NIDDM (2), gallbladder disease (7), sleep apnoea (8), and a number of cancers including breast cancer (9, 10) and colon cancer (11). In addition, further studies have shown a relationship between excess body weight and obstetric complications in women (12), progression of osteoarthritis (13), and rheumatoid arthritis (14).

There is a need for a comprehensive systematic review (e.g. a meta-analysis) to provide a clearer understanding of the relationships found in such studies between excess weight and the diseases. Once these data are available, relative risk estimates can be combined with country-specific overweight and obesity prevalence data to determine PAFs for use in cost-of-illness studies.

6.2.4 *The disability-adjusted life year*

An alternative to the cost-of-illness study for use in the economic evaluation of the consequences of obesity and overweight is the disability-adjusted life year (DALY) (*15*). This can provide estimates of the burden imposed by death and disability due to any disorder and makes it possible to compare populations in different geographical and social settings. Both the proportion of chronic diseases attributable to overweight and obesity and the costs of their management vary across populations and between social classes within populations. The use of a combined measure of the loss of life expectancy and prolonged morbidity in national, regional and global estimates of the economic effects of overweight and obesity is therefore desirable.

Obesity and overweight, in the same way as tobacco use, contribute to several NCDs. Thus, the total DALY loss attributable to obesity and overweight would represent the attributable fraction of the total loss of DALYs due to NCDs associated with excess body weight. A number of estimates of the attributable fraction associated with tobacco use have been made, thus facilitating national and regional comparisons. Efforts should therefore be made to generate similar estimates of the attributable fraction associated with obesity and overweight.

6.3 International estimates of the cost of obesity

6.3.1 *Studies in developed countries*

At present, the economic burden of obesity-related diseases has been estimated in only a few studies. Some of the data available for developed countries are reviewed below and summarized in Table 6.1. The scope and methodology of the various studies vary considerably in terms of the diseases costed, the definition of obesity, the cost

Table 6.1
Economic costs of obesity[a]

Country	Year	Study	BMI	Estimated direct costs	National health care costs
Australia	1989–1990	NHMRC (*16*)	>30	A$ 464 million	>2%
France	1992	Lévy et al. (*17*)	≥27	FF 12000 million	2%
Netherlands	1981–1989	Seidell & Deerenberg (*18*)	>25	NLG 1000 million	4%
USA	1994	Wolf & Colditz (*19*)	>29	US$ 45800 million	6.8%

[a] As defined by cut-off point of BMI.

categories used and the epidemiological assumptions as to the relationship between obesity and disease. This makes it difficult to compare costs across countries and to extrapolate the results from one country to another. The limited data available suggest that, as previously mentioned, some 2–7% of total health care expenditure in a country may be directly attributable to overweight and/or obesity.

Australia

The National Health and Medical Research Council (NHMRC) replicated the 1992 Colditz study (20), using the same obesity-related diseases and the same estimates of relative risk but applying Australian estimates of obesity prevalence (based on BMI >30). The NHMRC estimated the direct cost of obesity to be A$ 464 million (1989–1990), indirect costs amounting to an additional A$ 272 million. Hypertension and CHD combined accounted for approximately 60% of the total economic costs of obesity. For hypertension, the largest costs were those for medical services and pharmaceuticals, whereas for CHD, hospital costs and the indirect costs associated with premature mortality were the most significant (16).

As part of the total cost-of-obesity estimate, the NHMRC also estimated the costs of obesity treatment within the formal health care system in Australia. These accounted for approximately 10% of the total economic cost of obesity.

The estimate provided by the NHMRC should be considered conservative for the same reasons as the Colditz study in the USA. Of interest is the fact that, while the costs of obesity treatment within the health care sector amounted to less than A$ 80 million, a 1992 survey by the Consumer Advocacy and Financial Counselling Association of Victoria (21) estimated that 300000 consumers purchased a weight-loss programme in Australia each year from a variety of weight-loss centres, and that the industry turnover was in excess of A$ 500 million per annum. This shows that a substantial proportion of the economic cost of obesity is incurred outside the formal health care sector.

Finland

The impact of obesity on several indicators of health care utilization was assessed among 10000 adult Finns in the National Survey on Health and Social Security in 1987 (22). The costs of medicines, physician consultations and hospital inpatient stays increased with increasing BMI. The excess health care utilization was due mainly to an increased need for medication, the cost of which rose by about 12% when BMI increased from 25 to 40. On the basis of these data it was estimated that, if all Finns were of normal weight, the annual savings would be of the same order of magnitude as if all smokers in Finland were to stop smoking permanently.

France

To estimate the direct cost of obesity-related diseases in France in 1992, Lévy et al. (*17*) identified the direct costs of personal health care, hospital care, physician services and drugs for diseases with a well established relationship with obesity. These included NIDDM, hypertension, hyperlipidaemia, CHD, stroke, venous thromboembolism, osteoarthritis of the knee, gallbladder disease and certain cancers. The proportion of these diseases attributable to obesity (defined by the cut-off point of BMI ≥27) ranged from about 25% for hypertension and stroke to about 3% for breast cancer. The direct costs of obesity were estimated to be almost 12000 million francs, or approximately 2% of total health care expenditure in 1992. The costs of hypertension represented 53% of the total direct costs of obesity.

Netherlands

The cost of the excess use of medical care and associated costs due to obesity in the Netherlands were estimated using the data on 58000 participants in the Health Interview Surveys carried out from 1981 to 1989 (*18*). The health care costs included those for consultations with general practitioners and medical specialists, hospital admissions and the use of prescribed drugs. Obese (BMI ≥30) and overweight (BMI 25–30) individuals were more likely to have consulted a general practitioner. The total general practitioner costs attributable to obesity/overweight were equivalent to 3–4% of the country's total general practitioner expenditure. For hospitalizations, the fraction attributable to obesity was 3% and for overweight 2%. The excess use of medications by obese and overweight people, however, was very striking: compared with the non-obese, obese individuals were 5 times more likely to use diuretics and 2.5 times more likely to take drugs for CVD. It was estimated from these data that the direct costs of overweight and obesity were about 4% of total health care costs in the Netherlands. This is of the same order of magnitude as the health care costs attributable to all forms of cancer.

While the study did not cover all potential cost categories relevant to obesity, it was the first cost estimate to include the impact of overweight, and this category accounted for about 48% of the total costs of excess weight gain.

United States of America

The first national study undertaken on the economic cost of obesity was that by Colditz (*20*) in the USA. The diseases included in the cost estimate were NIDDM, CVD, hypertension, gallbladder disease, and colon and postmenopausal breast cancer. Obesity was defined as a BMI greater than 29. Total costs attributable to obesity in 1986, including both direct and indirect costs, were estimated to be US$ 39 300 million, representing 5.5% of the overall costs of illness for the USA in that year. The PAFs used for particular diseases were NIDDM 0.57, CVD 0.19, hypertension 0.26, breast cancer 0.06 and colon cancer 0.02. However, the estimates of relative risks used by Colditz are currently being revised by a number of groups to bring PAF and economic cost estimates into line with agreed classification criteria for overweight and obesity.

Colditz's original estimate should be considered conservative because estimates for many obesity-related diseases and for several relevant economic cost categories were excluded. Colditz points out that the addition of musculoskeletal disorders to his estimate would have raised the figure to US$ 56 300 million, or 7.8% of the cost of illness for the USA in 1986.

In 1994, Wolf & Colditz (*19*) published a revised estimate of the economic costs of obesity in the USA, extending the range of obesity-associated diseases included in the analysis and updating their calculations. They estimated that the total cost of obesity in 1990 was US$ 68 800 million, of which US$ 45 800 million was due to the direct cost of obesity-associated disease. The remaining US$ 23 300 million was an estimate of the indirect costs of obesity due to lost productivity (about US$ 4000 million, or 25 591 480 annual workdays) and premature mortality from diseases associated with obesity (about US$ 19 000 million). These figures should still be considered to be conservative.

6.3.2 *Studies on the broader economic issues*

Methods other than cost-of-illness studies have been used to determine the economic impact of obesity-related diseases, e.g. studies on the influence of obesity either on attainment of social class (see below) or on pension and disability payments.

It is important to note that indirect costs of disease relate to the loss of worker productivity due to worker absenteeism, staff turnover and reduced worker productivity as a result of obesity-related morbidity, together with lost earnings due to premature death from an obesity-related disease. A common misconception among health professionals is that sickness, unemployment and other social welfare benefits should be included in the indirect costs of diseases. Economists do not include such benefits in cost-of-illness studies as they are viewed as a transfer payment from the tax-paying population to the recipients. There is a continuing debate among health economists about whether to include indirect costs in a study and how to measure these costs reliably.

Attainment of social class

Cross-sectional studies in many affluent societies show an inverse relationship between educational level and the prevalence of obesity. However, in addition to indications that low socioeconomic status leads to obesity, there are also indications that the reverse may also be true. Obese subjects may also be subject to economic disadvantages such as higher premiums for life insurance policies.

One study of Danish draftees showed that, after adjustment for parental social class, level of education and intelligence, fewer obese men attained a relatively high social class compared with non-obese men (23). Similarly, a prospective study of young women in the USA showed that those who were obese were less likely to marry, and had fewer years of schooling, as well as a lower income compared with non-obese women (24). These results are supported by those of a number of other prospective studies showing that obese young adults do not attain the same social class as their non-obese peers. Although such data should be interpreted with caution, it has been suggested that societal discrimination may limit the socioeconomic potential of the obese.

Frequency of long-term sick-leave

In the SOS study (25) in Sweden, the frequency of long-term sick-leave (over 6 months) was reported to be 1.4 and 2.4 times higher in obese men and women, respectively, compared with the general Swedish population. Similarly, the rate of premature disability pensions was reported to be increased by a factor of 1.5–2.8 among participants in the study. The total loss of productivity due to obesity was estimated to be about 7% of the total cost of losses of productivity due to sick-leave and disability pensions in Sweden.

Premature work disability

In a large prospective Finnish study (26), obesity was associated with a twofold increased risk of premature work disability in men and a 1.5-fold greater risk in women. Most of the premature pensions attributable to obesity were due to cardiovascular and musculoskeletal diseases. A quarter of all disability pensions for these diseases in women were solely attributable to overweight and obesity.

6.3.3 *Studies in developing countries*

Although there have not been any comparable studies of the economic impact of obesity in developing countries, both WHO and the World Bank have recently highlighted the increasing burden associated with the rapidly emerging adult NCDs in these countries (*15, 27*), where they have now replaced infectious diseases as the leading cause of death. In developing countries, about 50% of deaths in 1990 were caused by NCDs, but by 2020 that proportion is expected to rise to almost 77%. In 1990, some 42% of deaths were attributed to infectious and reproductive conditions, while by 2020 that proportion is expected to decline to about 12%. In contrast, in developed countries 87% of deaths in 1990 were from NCDs and the proportion is expected to rise only slightly—to 90%—by 2020.

The treatment needs of the rapidly expanding urban populations and increasingly affluent middle classes in developing countries are already overwhelming many medical services. Furthermore, as previously mentioned, the real costs of therapy associated with NCDs in developing countries exceed those in developed countries; the need to use scarce foreign exchange to pay for imports of expensive equipment and drugs and for the training of specialized staff creates an extra burden.

In recent World Bank studies, e.g. in Chile (*28*), the burden of disease has been expressed in terms of numbers of DALYs lost. NCDs account for a 5- and 9-fold greater rate of premature death than communicable diseases in men and women, respectively, and 10- and 5-fold greater rates of disability. The numbers of DALYs lost in men are 15-fold, and in women 20-fold, greater for NCDs than for infections. So far, the burden of disease attributable to excess weight gain and obesity has not been calculated, but cancers impose a substantial burden as do NIDDM and CVD. There is thus a need in developing countries to apply the new economic methods of determining the proportion of these diseases attributable to excess weight gain so that the impact of one of the principal contributors to NCDs can be assessed.

6.3.4 *Conclusions*

International studies on the economic costs of obesity have shown that they account for between 2% and 7% of total health care costs, the level depending on the range of diseases and cost categories included in the analysis. The figures are based mainly on cross-sectional data, and should be considered a conservative estimate of the true cost of obesity-related diseases for a number of reasons:

- In most studies, only a limited number of obesity-related diseases have been costed.

- Most studies have excluded some relevant direct-cost categories from the analysis.

- In the majority of cases only the economic costs associated with obesity (BMI ≥30) have been included in the analysis. The inclusion of costs associated with overweight (i.e. BMI 25–29.9) would substantially increase the attributed cost because the number of overweight individuals in a community is generally greater by a factor of 3–4 than those who are obese; the economic cost of drug use, for example, was increased by 65% if the overweight category was included (*18*).

Although there have not been any comparable studies of the economic impact of obesity in developing countries, the real costs of therapy associated with NCDs in such countries are likely to exceed those in developed countries.

6.4 Economic costs and benefits of obesity treatment

6.4.1 *Analyses of obesity-control trials*

Unfortunately, very little information is available on the economic benefits of treatment, but some extrapolations can be made from the preliminary and early data from the large-scale SOS intervention study of 1743 obese men and women in Sweden (*25*).

After 2 years of follow-up, Sjöström and his colleagues found a number of benefits in the subjects who were surgically treated and who individually lost between 30 kg and 40 kg. Thus quality of life was markedly improved and several cardiovascular risk factors were substantially decreased. The prevalence of NIDDM — 13% in controls and 16% in the intervention group before treatment — decreased by 68% in the intervention group and by only 16% in the controls. In other words, two-thirds of NIDDM was "cured" by the obesity intervention. Furthermore, the incidence of NIDDM was only 0.5% in the intervention group as compared with 7% in the controls. A 4–5-fold risk reduction was observed in the development of hypertension, hypertriglyceridaemia and the lowering of HDL cholesterol. During 2 years of follow-up, the incidence of NIDDM was very low in the intervention group but 30-fold higher in controls. Data on other disease end-points are not yet available.

In order to try to estimate the economic consequences of this controlled study, the results of treatment and the associated costs may be compared with the estimated costs of non-treated obese subjects. If

NIDDM is taken as an example, the 14-fold risk reduction in the treatment group suggests that NIDDM was prevented to a large extent. In addition, two-thirds of patients with established NIDDM were "cured". Applying these results to the estimated cost of obesity-related NIDDM in France would decrease the total costs of obesity in that country by approximately 3%, while in the USA costs could be reduced by almost 20%. Similar calculations with respect to change in cardiovascular risk factors are not easy, but a large proportion of the obese subjects who would usually be eligible for treatment for hypertension and hyperlipidaemia would not need such treatment. In France this would result in a 25% reduction in costs.

Little published information is so far available on the potential impact of obesity treatment in the SOS trial on sick-leave and pensions, which constitute the other major component of the costs of obesity. This is difficult to evaluate because treated patients have not been followed up for a long enough period, but the initial data indicated that the number of lost working days increased more quickly in the controls than in the intervention groups (25). Furthermore, the marked improvements in the quality of life of treated patients are not only an important outcome in themselves but also suggest that other major benefits that would reduce health costs can be expected after longer follow-up.

However, it is important to include in the costs those of the intervention itself (i.e. surgery) and of the follow-up review. The actual cost of the surgical procedure is not available, but follow-up figures suggest that, in spite of the surgical intervention, the frequency of visits to a doctor was the same in controls and intervention subjects by the second year after surgery.

The SOS study is the only fully controlled, large-scale, long-term study of the effects of the radical treatment of obesity and substantial weight loss. The results of this study will provide valuable information on the medical and economic consequences of effective intervention in obesity within a limited period. Preliminary results are very promising.

6.4.2 Potential cost savings associated with a reduction in the prevalence of obesity

A small number of studies have provided estimates of the potential impact on health care costs of a reduction in the population prevalence of obesity.

In a study in the USA (29), obese patients with NIDDM were assigned to a 12-week weight-loss programme involving an 800-kcal$_{th}$

diet (1 kcal$_{th}$ = 4.18 kJ). Subjects lost an average of 15.3 kg over the 12 weeks, but at 1-year follow-up had regained 9.0 kg. The authors estimated that the average saving in prescription costs per subject over 1 year was US$ 442.80. While the study showed a significant prescription cost saving, sample sizes were small and the energy intake associated with the weight-loss programme was very small. It would thus be unwise to assume that these results would be reproduced under different conditions.

As an extension of a cost-of-obesity study discussed earlier in this section (see p. 84), the NHMRC estimated the potential annual saving to the Australian health care system that would result if the prevalence of obesity were reduced by 20% by the year 2000 (baseline 1989), as specified by the National Health Goals and Targets (30). The method used in this study was to recalculate the PAF based on the target prevalence of obesity (and on the assumption that relative risk estimates remain constant) for each obesity-related disease. The 1989–1990 estimated cost for each obesity-related disease was then multiplied by the change in PAF to estimate the potential annual saving. The NHMRC estimated that an annual saving of A$ 59 million in health care expenditure and a potential 2300 life-years could be gained if the obesity target was achieved.

While the NHMRC calculation shows the potential cost saving that might be achieved if the target obesity prevalence were achieved, it does not provide information on the public and private expenditure that would be required to fund programmes to achieve this target. The analysis therefore does not help decision-makers to decide whether investing scarce community resources in preventing or treating overweight and obesity represents an efficient use of such resources. Such decisions should be based on an evaluation of the costs and outcomes (effectiveness) of alternative interventions for the prevention and treatment of overweight and obesity.

6.4.3 *Cost–effectiveness of obesity prevention and treatment*

Few studies have addressed the economic evaluation of the prevention and treatment of overweight and obesity and, of these, most have been concerned with treatment rather than primary prevention. A limited number of studies on the cost-effectiveness of non-drug versus drug treatment of hypertension have been conducted and have included measurements of weight loss. In addition, a number of studies have focused on the financial benefits of workplace fitness programmes (including the benefit of weight loss) in reducing employee absenteeism, but the methods used in these studies have been criticized (31, 32). Authors have sometimes overgeneralized and used optimistic estimates of the health benefits of risk factor modification. In other studies, the relevant programme cost categories have been incorrectly specified, and rather dubious methods of valuing and measuring these costs have been used. The results seem in some instances to be biased in favour of finding workplace health promotion to be a good investment.

The results of two studies on the cost–effectiveness of alternative interventions for weight control are discussed below.

Cost–effectiveness of obesity management in the prevention of NIDDM
In a recent study by Segal et al. (*33*), an attempt was made to model the potential cost–effectiveness of a range of interventions for the prevention and treatment of NIDDM in Australia. These interventions included a population approach using mass media programmes focusing on lifestyle changes (including diet and exercise); a behaviour modification programme for the seriously obese; a group programme targeting overweight men (based on an established programme called GutBusters); gastric surgery for the morbidly obese; and a behaviour modification programme for women who had gestational NIDDM.

Both the costs and outcomes of the various interventions were estimated. Net costs (or savings) were derived by adding together programme costs and the potential savings in future health care costs from the prevention of cases of NIDDM. Outcomes were expressed as NIDDM years deferred and life-years saved. Costs were based on reports in the literature, discussions with service providers and published health service cost data. Epidemiological data reported in the literature were used in assessing the effectiveness of various programmes in preventing NIDDM. A range of estimates was calculated based on different assumptions as to programme success, programme costs and other important variables.

The most cost-effective interventions were found to be the GutBusters Programme (a commercial 6-week group session programme for men) and the mass media lifestyle modification programme. It was estimated that both would lead to future cost savings resulting from the reduced incidence of NIDDM, and these savings would be greater than the programme costs. Table 6.2 summarizes the main results of the study.

Although the results presented in Table 6.2 depend very much on the assumption of long-term success in the various weight-loss programmes, the wide range of cost–effectiveness estimates indicate that they are robust. Indeed, while the analysis incorporates the esti-

Table 6.2
Summary of the estimated cost–effectiveness of a range of interventions for the prevention of NIDDM[a]

Intervention[a]	Net cost per NIDDM year avoided (A$)	Net cost per life-year gained (A$)
Surgery for seriously obese:		
all IGT[b]	1 200	4 600
10% IGT, 90% normal[c]	3 500	12 300
Diet/behaviour modification for seriously obese:		
all IGT	saving	saving
10% IGT, 90% normal	1 600	2 600
Group programme for overweight men:		
all IGT	saving	saving
10% IGT, 90% normal	saving	saving
Diet/behavioural programme for women with previous gestational NIDDM:		
all IGT	800	1 200
30% IGT, 70% normal	2 100	2 400
Media programme	saving	saving

[a] Reproduced from reference 33 with the permission of the publisher.
[b] "IGT" refers to programmes targeted at those with impaired glucose tolerance.
[c] "normal" relates to normal glucose tolerance.

mated effect of weight loss on all-cause mortality, and not just that associated with NIDDM, the probable impact of a successful prevention programme on other risk factors (such as cholesterol or blood pressure) has not been taken into account. In addition, the expected savings in future health care costs relate to NIDDM only, ignoring possible savings in the management of other obesity-related diseases. For these reasons the results may well be conservative.

The authors of the study concluded that the prevention of NIDDM, through appropriate interventions, can represent a highly efficient use of community resources. Such programmes can achieve a substantial improvement in health status at little cost or indeed with the possibility of a net saving in the use of health care resources.

Cost–effectiveness of commercial weight-loss programmes
A study by Spielman et al. (*34*) analysed the cost of losing weight in commercial weight-loss programmes in the Boston metropolitan area. It reviewed 11 commercial diet programmes and estimated for each programme the out-of-pocket cost to the participant (over a 12-week

period) of losing 1 kg. The diet programmes were divided into three groups:

1. Medically supervised very-low-calorie diets (VLCDs) that provide <800 kcal$_{th}$/per day.[1]
2. Nutrient-balance reduced-energy diet programmes (REDPs), the client consuming 800–1200 kcal$_{th}$/day[1] (50% carbohydrate, 15–20% protein, <30% fat).
3. Support groups that may or may not offer individual dietary advice and act as a self-help programme with volunteer staff.

It was found that the cost of a 12-week commercial weight-loss programme varied enormously, from US$ 2120 for the most expensive VLCD to US$ 108 for the least expensive REDP. The data are summarized in Table 6.3.

This short-term analysis suggests that support groups and lower-cost REDPs were the most cost-effective interventions. Dietitians were only marginally better value for money than REDPs, particularly when the expected reduction in usual supermarket expenditures is subtracted. However, the study can be criticized on a number of grounds:

- Weight loss in a sample of programme participants was not measured. Instead, the "expected" weight loss based on the literature was used and excellent compliance was assumed throughout the duration of the programme. Weight loss may thus be substantially overestimated and in practice there would be significant differences in the weight loss achieved by the different programmes. Potential drop-out rates are also ignored.

- The study was based on a 12-week programme, did not take into account the costs and impacts of weight-maintenance programmes, and could not take account of the longer-term impact of the competing programmes.

- The financial "costs" measured were restricted to programme initiation fees, the cost of any food supplements purchased as a result of the programme (e.g. liquid protein formulae for VLCDs, or preprepared foods for REDPs) and of medical monitoring and/or associated behaviour modification programmes. Additional costs (or savings) associated with daily food purchases, reduced-energy beverages, etc., were not taken into account. Thus, for a

---

[1] 1 kcal$_{th}$ = 4.18 kJ.

Table 6.3
Cost in US$ per kilogram of active weight loss (12 weeks)[a]

Programme type	Initial weight	
	80 kg	136 kg
Nutrient-balanced REDP:		
Jenny Craig	23.00	13.50
Nutri-System	19.00	12.00
Registered dietitian	15.00	9.00
Weight Watchers	2.50	1.50
VLCD programmes:		
Health Management Resources (HMR)	17.50	10.00
Medifast	14.00	8.00
Support groups:		
Taking Off Pounds Sensibly (TOPS)	0.07	0.04

[a] Reproduced from reference 34 with the permission of the publisher.

commercial programme, the cost of prepared food plus additional staple items purchased from the supermarket have to be compared with usual food bills.

• The "time" costs of attending the programmes were also not taken into account. These costs may be significant and would differ from one programme to another.

If all the costs had been included and the effectiveness of the interventions measured, the costs of the programmes might well have been different.

Economic costs and benefits of obesity treatment in developing countries
No analyses have been made of the economic costs of obesity treatment in developing countries. However, other analyses of the costs of health interventions show that prevention is more cost-effective than treatment once disease is diagnosed. In Table 6.4, the costs of a variety of public health packages (including education, information, surveillance and monitoring) are compared with those of some primary care clinical services in developing countries where the major needs are the treatment of trauma and infection. Low-income developing countries do not have the resources to provide anything other than public health and essential clinical services. In middle-income developing countries, the high costs of discretionary clinical services (see Table 6.4) mean that the cost of dealing with chronic diseases exceeds that of all other forms of health care. Thus, it would appear to be more cost-effective for money spent on obesity and other NCDs to

Table 6.4
Allocation of public expenditure on health in developing countries, 1990[a]

Type of service	Allocation in developing countries (US$ per person per year)[b]		Contents of health-related packages	Cost per DALY (US$)
	Actual	Proposed		
Public health package	1	5	Immunizations; school health programmes; tobacco and alcohol control; health, nutrition and family planning information; vector control; STD prevention; monitoring and surveillance.	25
Essential clinical services	4–6[c]	10	Treatment of tuberculosis, STDs; infection and minor trauma; management of the sick child; prenatal and delivery care; family planning; assessment, advice, and minor pain alleviation.	25–75
Discretionary clinical services[d]	13–15	6	All other health services, including low-cost treatment of cancer, CVD, other chronic conditions, major trauma, and neurological and psychiatric disorders.	>1000
Total	21	21		

[a] Source: references 35 and 36.
[b] Estimates are for all developing countries, i.e. an average of costs in low-income countries (annual income US$ 350 per capita) and middle-income countries (annual income US$ 2500 per capita). The figures shown should be regarded as approximate.
[c] Based on estimates in World Bank health sector reports, current spending on essential clinical services is estimated to be 20–30% of total public expenditure on health.
[d] Estimated as total cost of overall health packages minus cost of public health and essential clinical services packages.

be used for prevention rather than for expensive treatments during the advanced stage of disease.

Public health action to prevent obesity has the added benefit of involving the establishment of new or improved physical and social structures within a community, many of which can have long-term positive effects for both current and future generations. Treatment systems, however, are likely to demand recurrent expenditure as new cases of obesity emerge, together with the need for either long-term or repeated treatment. At present, most individuals with excess weight gain in developing countries are not treated, and the demand for medical and dietetic help is expected to rise rapidly. In addition, limited resources will be diverted to pay for slimming diets and other aids to weight loss.

In developing countries where NCD epidemics are emerging or accelerating, a large proportion of NCD deaths occur in the productive middle years of life, at ages much younger than those seen in developed countries. The health burdens attributable to excess weight gain in societies in transition are likely to be huge because of the absolute numbers at risk, the large reduction in life expectancy and the fact that the problem affects, in particular, individuals with a key role in promoting economic development.

References

1. Davey PJ, Leeder SR. The cost of cost-of-illness studies. *Medical Journal of Australia*, 1993, **158**:583–584.

2. Perry IJ et al. Prospective study of risk factors for development of non-insulin-dependent diabetes in middle-aged British men. *British Medical Journal*, 1995, **310**:560–564.

3. Rimm EB et al. Body size and fat distribution as predictors of coronary heart disease among middle-aged and older US men. *American Journal of Epidemiology*, 1995, **141**:1117–1127.

4. Walker M. Weight change and risk of heart attack in middle-aged British men. *International Journal of Epidemiology*, 1995, **24**:694–703.

5. MacMahon SO et al. Blood pressure, stroke, and coronary heart disease. Part I, Prolonged differences in blood pressure: prospective observational studies corrected for the regression dilution bias. *Lancet*, 1990, **335**:765–774.

6. Abbott RD et al. Body mass index and thromboembolic stroke in nonsmoking men in older middle age. The Honolulu Heart Program. *Stroke*, 1994, **25**:2370–2376.

7. La Vecchia C et al. Risk factors for gallstone disease requiring surgery. *International Journal of Epidemiology*, 1991, **20**:209–215.

8. Carlson JT et al. High prevalence of hypertension in sleep apnea patients independent of obesity. *American Journal of Respiratory and Critical Care Medicine*, 1994, **150**:72–77.

9. Zhang S et al. Better breast cancer survival for postmenopausal women who are less overweight and eat less fat. The Iowa Women's Health Study. *Cancer*, 1995, **76**:275–283.

10. Yong LC et al. Prospective study of relative weight and risk of breast cancer: the Breast Cancer Detection Demonstration Project follow-up study, 1979 to 1987–89. *American Journal of Epidemiology*, 1996, **143**:985–995.

11. Giovannucci E et al. Physical activity, obesity and risk for colon cancer and adenoma in men. *Annals of Internal Medicine*, 1995, **122**:327–334.

12. Siega-Riz AM, Adair LS, Hobel CJ. Institute of Medicine maternal weight gain recommendations and pregnancy outcome in a predominantly Hispanic population. *Obstetrics and Gynecology*, 1994, **84**:565–573.

13. Spector TD, Hart DJ, Doyle DV. Incidence and progression of osteoarthritis in women with unilateral knee disease in the general population: the effect of obesity. *Annals of the Rheumatic Diseases*, 1994, **53**:565–568.

14. Voigt LF et al. Smoking, obesity, alcohol consumption, and the risk of rheumatoid arthritis. *Epidemiology*, 1994, **5**:525–532.

15. Murray CJL, Lopez AD, eds. *The global burden of disease*. Boston, MA, Harvard University Press, 1996.

16. National Health and Medical Research Council. Economic issues in the prevention and treatment of overweight and obesity. In: *Acting on Australia's weight: a strategic plan for the prevention of overweight and obesity*. Canberra, Australian Government Publishing Service, 1997:85–95.

17. Lévy E et al. The economic cost of obesity: the French situation. *International Journal of Obesity and Related Metabolic Disorders*, 1995, **19**:788–792.

18. Seidell J, Deerenberg I. Obesity in Europe — prevalence and consequences for the use of medical care. *PharmacoEconomics*, 1994, **5**(Suppl. 1):38–44.

19. Wolf AM, Colditz GA. The costs of obesity: the U.S. perspective. *PharmacoEconomics*, 1994, **5**:34–37.

20. Colditz GA. Economic costs of obesity. *American Journal of Clinical Nutrition*, 1992, **55**(2 Suppl.):503S–507S.

21. *Tipping the scales*. Melbourne, The Consumer Advocacy and Financial Counselling Association of Australia, 1992.

22. Häkkinen U. The production of health and the demand for health care in Finland. *Social Science and Medicine*, 1991, **33**:225–237.

23. Sonne-Holm S, Sorensen TI. Prospective study of attainment of social class of severely obese subjects in relation to parental social class, intelligence and education. *British Medical Journal*, 1986, **292**:586–589.

24. Gortmaker SL et al. Social and economic consequences of overweight in adolescence and young adulthood. *New England Journal of Medicine*, 1993, **329**:1008–1012.

25. Sjöström L, Narbro K, Sjöström D. Costs and benefits when treating obesity. *International Journal of Obesity and Related Metabolic Disorders*, 1995, **19**(Suppl. 6):S9–S12.

26. Rissanen A et al. Risk of disability and mortality due to overweight in a Finnish population. *British Medical Journal*, 1990, **301**:835–837.

27. *The World Health Report, 1997. Conquering suffering, enriching humanity*. Geneva, World Health Organization, 1997.

28. *Chile: the adult health policy challenge.* Washington, DC, World Bank, 1995 (World Bank Country Study Series).

29. **Collins RW, Anderson JW.** Medication cost savings associated with weight loss for obese non-insulin-dependent diabetic men and women. *Preventive Medicine,* 1995, **24**:369–374.

30. *National health strategy: pathways to better health.* Canberra, Department of Health, Housing and Community Services, March 1993 (Issues Paper no. 7).

31. **Shephard RJ.** Current perspectives on the economics of fitness and sport with particular reference to worksite programs. *Sports Medicine,* 1989, **7**:286–309.

32. **Shephard RJ.** A critical analysis of work-site fitness programs and their postulated economic benefits. *Medicine and Science in Sports and Exercise,* 1992, **24**:354–370.

33. **Segal L, Dalton A, Richardson J.** *The cost-effectiveness of primary prevention for non-insulin-dependent diabetes mellitus.* Melbourne, Health Economics Unit, Faculty of Business and Economics, Monash University, 1997 (Centre for Health Program Evaluation, Research Report 8).

34. **Spielman AB et al.** The cost of losing: an analysis of commercial weight-loss programs in a metropolitan area. *Journal of the American College of Nutrition,* 1992, **11**:36–41.

35. **World Bank.** *World Development Report 1993: Investing in health: world development indicators.* New York, Oxford University Press, 1993.

36. *Food, nutrition and the prevention of cancer: a global perspective.* Washington, DC, World Cancer Research Fund/American Institute for Cancer Research, 1997.

PART III

Understanding how overweight and obesity develop

7. Factors influencing the development of overweight and obesity

7.1 Introduction

In simple terms, obesity is a consequence of an energy imbalance — energy intake exceeds energy expenditure over a considerable period. Many complex and diverse factors can give rise to a positive energy balance, but it is the interaction between a number of these factors, rather than the influence of any single factor, that is thought to be responsible. In contrast to the widely held perception among the public and parts of the scientific and medical communities, it is clear that obesity is not simply a result of overindulgence in highly palatable foods, or of a lack of physical activity.

The various influences on energy intake and expenditure that are considered to be important in weight gain and the development of obesity are considered below. Section 7.2 gives an overview of the fundamental principles of energy balance, the physiological regulation of body weight and the dynamics of weight gain. Section 7.3 examines the role of dietary factors and physical activity patterns in weight gain. Section 7.4 discusses the multitude of environmental and societal forces that adversely affect food intake and physical activity patterns, and may thus overwhelm the normal regulatory processes that control the long-term energy balance. Finally, section 7.5 reviews the various genetic, physiological or medical factors that can determine an individual's susceptibility to those forces and that put that person at higher risk of weight gain and obesity.

The following should be noted:

- Obesity can result from a minor energy imbalance that leads to a gradual but persistent weight gain over a considerable period. Once the obese state is established, physiological processes tend to maintain the new weight.

- Body weight is primarily regulated by a series of physiological processes but is also influenced by external societal and cognitive factors.

- Recent epidemiological trends in obesity indicate that the primary cause of the global obesity problem lies in environmental and behavioural changes. The rapid increase in obesity rates has occurred in too short a time for there to have been significant genetic changes within populations.

- The increasing proportion of fat and the increased energy density of the diet, together with reductions in the level of physical activity and the rise in that of sedentary behaviour, are thought to be major contributing factors to the rise in the average body weight of populations. Dealing with these issues would appear to be the most effective means of combating rises in the level of overweight and obesity in the community.

- The global obesity problem can be viewed as a consequence of the massive social, economic and cultural problems now facing developing and newly industrialized countries, as well as ethnic minorities and the disadvantaged in developed countries. Escalating rates of obesity, NIDDM, hypertension, dyslipidaemia and CVD, coupled with cigarette smoking and alcohol abuse, are frequent outcomes of the modernization/acculturation process.

- Epidemiological, genetic and molecular studies in many populations of the world suggest that there are people who are more susceptible to weight gain and the development of obesity than others. Genetic, biological and other personal factors such as smoking cessation, sex and age interact to determine an individual's susceptibility to weight gain.

- Certain ethnic groups appear to be especially liable to the development of obesity when exposed to an affluent lifestyle, although susceptibilities to obesity comorbidities are not uniform across these groups.

7.2 Energy balance and the physiological regulation of body weight

The major influences on energy balance and weight gain are shown in Fig. 7.1.

7.2.1 Fundamental principles of energy balance

The fundamental principle of energy balance is:

changes in energy stores = energy intake − energy expenditure

A positive energy balance occurs when energy intake is greater than energy expenditure; it promotes an increase in energy stores and body weight. Conversely, a negative energy balance occurs when intake is less than expenditure, promoting a decrease in energy stores and body weight.

Under normal circumstances, the energy balance oscillates from meal to meal, day to day and week to week without any lasting change in body stores or weight. Multiple physiological mechanisms act within each individual to equate overall energy intake with overall energy expenditure and to keep body weight stable in the long term. Thus, it

Figure 7.1
Influences on energy balance and weight gain (energy regulation)

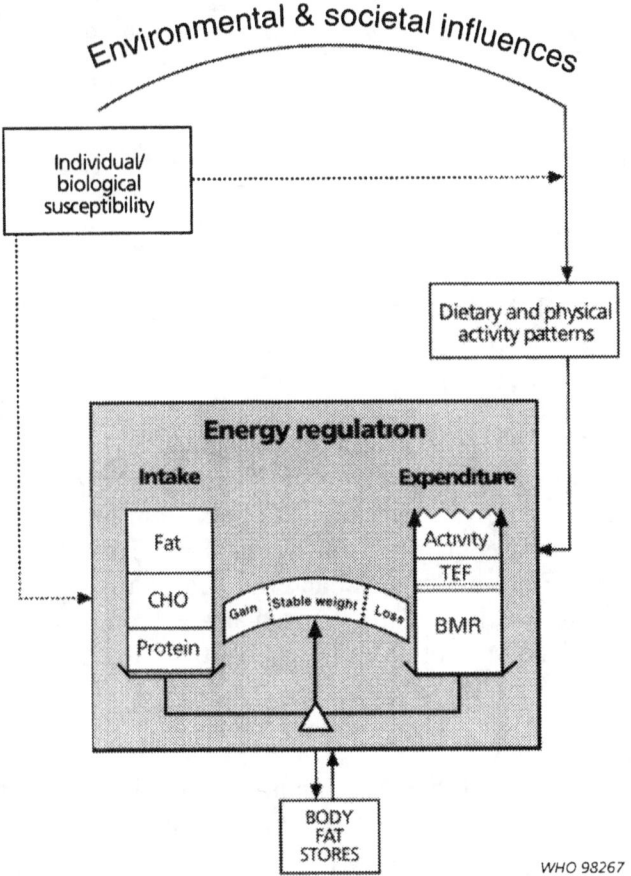

WHO 98267

The diagram shows the fundamental principles of energy balance and regulation. A positive energy balance occurs when energy intake is greater than energy expenditure, and promotes weight gain. Conversely, a negative energy balance promotes a decrease in body fat stores and weight loss. Body weight is regulated by a series of physiological processes that have the capacity to maintain weight within a relatively narrow range (stable weight). It is thought that the body exerts a stronger defence against undernutrition and weight loss than it does against overconsumption and weight gain. However, powerful societal and environmental forces influence energy intake and expenditure, and may overwhelm the above-mentioned physiological processes. The susceptibility of individuals to these forces is affected by genetic and other biological factors, such as sex, age and hormonal activities, over which they have little or no control. Dietary factors and physical activity patterns are considered to be the modifiable intermediate factors through which the forces that promote weight gain act.

TEF = thermic effect of food; BMR = basal metabolic rate; CHO = carbohydrate.

Table 7.1
Energy content of macronutrients

Macronutrient	Energy contribution	
	(kcal$_{th}$/g)	(kJ/g)
Fat	9	37
Alcohol	7	29
Protein	4	17
Carbohydrate	4	16

is only when there has been a positive energy balance for a considerable period that obesity is likely to develop.

Energy intake
Total energy intake refers to all energy consumed as food and drink that can be metabolized inside the body. Table 7.1 shows the energy content of the constituent macronutrients present in food and drink. Fat provides the most energy per unit weight, and carbohydrate and protein the least. Fibre undergoes bacterial degradation in the large intestine to produce volatile fatty acids that are then absorbed and used as energy. The size of the energy contribution from fibre is thought to be 6.3 kJ/g (1.5 kcal$_{th}$/g) (*1*).

Energy expenditure
The second element of the energy balance equation, total energy expenditure, has the following three main components:

— the basal metabolic rate (BMR);
— dietary thermogenesis (meal-induced heat production);
— physical activity.

The proportion that each component contributes to the total energy expenditure varies according to the regularity and intensity of physical activity. In sedentary adults, the BMR accounts for nearly 60% of total energy output, the dietary thermogenic response for around 10%, and physical activity for the remaining 30%. In those engaged in heavy manual work, total energy expenditure increases and the proportion of energy expenditure accounted for by physical activity may rise to about 50%. Dietary thermogenesis appears to remain constant at 10%, leaving the BMR to account for 40% of the total energy expenditure. Although the BMR may vary intrinsically between individuals of similar weight by ±25%, within each individual it is tightly controlled (*2*). The key variable of energy output in an individual is the degree of physical activity.

7.2.2 *Physiological regulation of body weight*

Societal and cognitive factors can influence the control of body weight to a certain extent, but it is a series of physiological processes that are primarily responsible for body weight regulation. In traditional societies, where people tend to be more physically active, and provided that food supplies are not limited, few adults are either underweight or overweight despite the interaction of seasonal cycles of work, festivities, individual susceptibilities to obesity for physiological or genetic reasons, and the wide range of varying physical demands within a society. Such physiological mechanisms constitute a fundamentally important biological process that can be observed throughout the animal kingdom. It is thought that the body exerts a stronger defence against undernutrition and weight loss than it does against overconsumption and weight gain (3).

The physiological mechanisms responsible for body weight regulation are incompletely understood. However, there is increasing evidence of a range of signalling mechanisms within the intestine, the adipose tissue and brain, and perhaps within other tissues, that sense the inflow of dietary nutrients, their distribution and metabolism and/or storage. These mechanisms are coordinated within the brain and lead to changes in eating, in physical activity and in body metabolism so that body energy stores are maintained. The recent discovery of the hormone leptin, which is secreted by adipocytes in proportion to their triglyceride stores and binds with receptors in the hypothalamus, provides interesting insights into possible regulatory signal systems that act to maintain the energy balance. However, much remains to be elucidated about such systems, some of which are illustrated in Fig. 7.2.

7.2.3 *Dynamics of weight gain*

Despite the extensive physiological regulation of body weight outlined above, a positive energy balance can lead to weight gain if it persists in the long term. The initiation of a chronic positive energy balance is due to an increase in energy intake relative to requirements, either as a result of an increase in total energy intake, a decrease in total energy expenditure, or a combination of the two. Currently there is little information about the fluctuations in energy balance that lead to weight gain and obesity. It is possible that large deviations from energy balance at regular intervals may contribute to weight gain, but it is believed that a small consistent deviation over a long period is also capable of producing large increases in body weight.

Figure 7.2

Physiological processes involved in body weight regulation

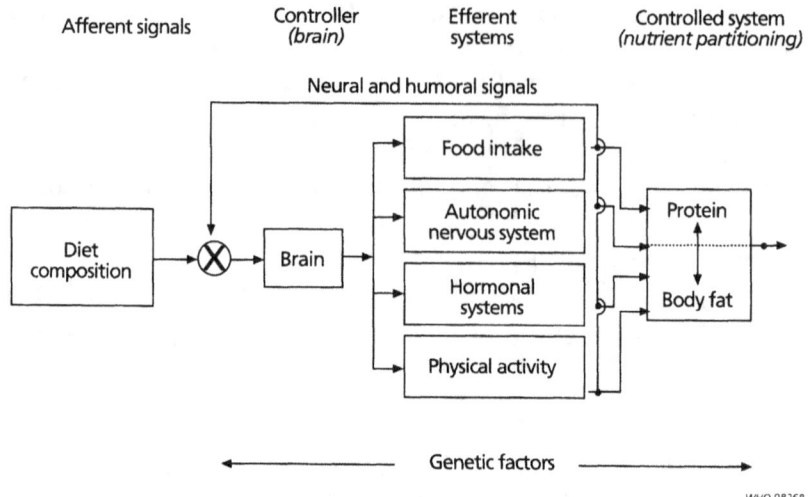

WHO 98268

The diagram shows the interaction between the different mechanisms that affect energy and body weight regulation within individuals. The brain integrates an array of afferent signals (nutrient, metabolic, hormonal and neuronal) and responds by inducing changes in food intake, autonomic nervous system activity, hormonal responses or spontaneous physical activity. The different components then directly or indirectly determine the proportion of dietary energy deposited as protein rather than fat.

Fig. 7.3 shows that the process of gaining weight can be divided into the following three phases:

- The *preobese static phase*, when the individual is in long-term energy balance and weight remains constant.

- The *dynamic phase*, during which the individual gains weight as a result of energy intake exceeding energy expenditure over a prolonged period.

- The *obese static phase*, when energy balance is regained but weight is now higher than during the preobese static phase.

The dynamic phase can last for several years and often involves considerable fluctuations in weight (weight cycling) as a result of conscious efforts by the individual to return to a lower weight. However, in the absence of intervention, the difference between energy intake and energy expenditure progressively diminishes. This is due to an increase in BMR as a result of the larger fat-free mass (including that in the expanded adipose tissue) as well as to an additional energy

Figure 7.3
**Effect on energy expenditure, energy balance and body weight of an increase in
energy intake relative to requirements[a]**

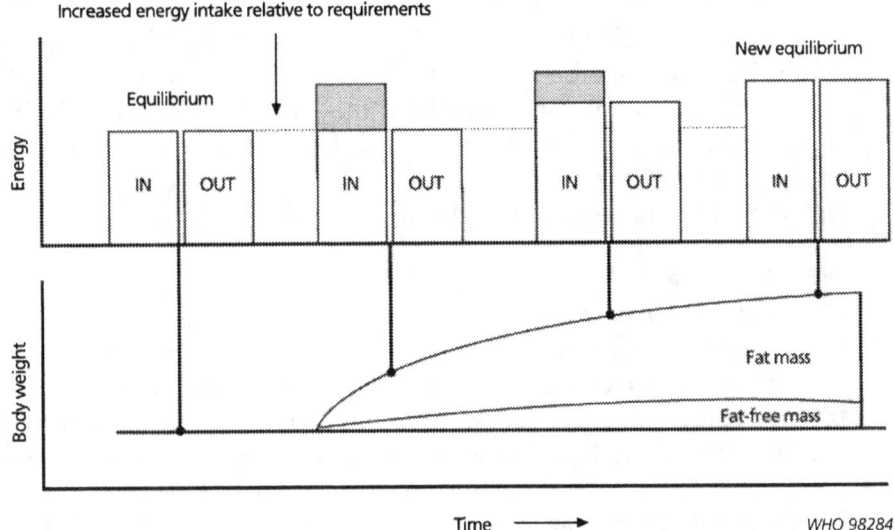

A persistent increase in energy intake above requirements will lead to a gradual gain in body
weight. However, the size of the energy imbalance progressively diminishes as weight is
gained, because of an increase in metabolism associated with the larger fat-free mass and the
expanded adipose tissue. A new higher equilibrium weight is eventually established that is
again defended by physiological mechanisms. Thus, it is harder to lose the weight gained than
it is to experience a second cycle of increasing body weight should, for example, a fall in
physical activity occur at the same time as a further period of prolonged positive energy
balance.

[a] Adapted, with permission, from: Schutz Y. Macronutrients and energy balance in obesity.
Metabolism, 1995, 4(9 Suppl. 3):7–11 (reference 4).

cost of activity imposed by the extra weight (5). There may also be an
increase in resting metabolic rate (RMR) with overfeeding (6).

Once the obese static phase is established, the new weight appears to
be defended. This can best be shown by the response of obese individuals to underfeeding; they show a fall in metabolic rate as the body
recognizes the loss of energy (7) and an unconscious physiologically
driven increase in energy intake (8).

7.2.4 *Implications for public health*

Given the global epidemic of obesity, the aim should be:

— to identify the environmental factors, including societal changes,
that have overwhelmed the physiological regulatory processes
outlined above;

— to determine whether some individuals are more susceptible to those influences for medical, behavioural or genetic reasons.

7.3 Dietary factors and physical activity patterns

Dietary factors and physical activity patterns strongly influence the energy balance equation and can be considered to be the major modifiable factors through which many of the external forces promoting weight gain act (Fig. 7.1). In particular, high-fat, energy-dense diets and sedentary lifestyles are the two characteristics most strongly associated with the increased prevalence of obesity worldwide.

7.3.1 Dietary factors

Macronutrient composition

Laboratory experiments in animals and clinical studies in humans have repeatedly shown that dietary factors, particularly the level of fat and energy intake, are strongly and positively associated with excess body weight. By contrast, population-based studies of diet and obesity have reported inconsistent results. Such inconsistencies have been attributed to a number of factors, including weaknesses in study design, methodological flaws, confounders, and random and/or systematic measurement error in the data, especially the dietary data (9). Thus, in population studies that pay careful attention to the determinants of obesity, a positive association is observed between dietary factors and obesity identical with those found in animal models and human clinical studies (10).

Energy intake. Dietary fat has a higher energy density than other macronutrients (see Table 7.1, p. 104 and Table 7.2, p. 111). This is thought to be largely responsible for the overeating effect, or *passive overconsumption* as it is often called, experienced by many subjects exposed to high-fat foods (3). The stimulatory effect of fatty foods on energy intake may also be due to the pleasant mouth-feel of fat when eaten (11).

The body does compensate for the overconsumption of energy from high-fat foods to some extent, but the fat-induced appetite control signals are thought to be too weak, or too delayed, to prevent the rapid intake of the energy from a fatty meal. Episodic intakes of high-fat foods are therefore particularly likely to overwhelm these signals, and the control of food intake thus depends on long-term regulatory processes that seem much less able to respond to overfeeding than to underfeeding with weight loss. Fibre, by contrast, limits energy intake by lowering a food's density and allowing time for appetite-control signals to occur before large amounts of energy have been consumed (3).

There is no clear evidence to suggest that high intakes of sugar overwhelm the appetite-control signals in the same manner as fat. However, there is some indication from short-term feeding trials that *ad libitum* low-fat high-complex-carbohydrate diets of low energy density induce weight loss. This does not occur on energy-dense diets, regardless of whether the energy density has been increased by modifying the fat content or the sugar content of the diet (*12*). Further studies are required before any conclusions can be drawn from this work.

Energy storage and macronutrient balance. The macronutrient composition of the diet also influences the extent to which excess energy is stored, depending on the storage capacity within the body of the macronutrients concerned, those macronutrients with a low storage capacity within the body being preferentially oxidized when intakes exceed requirements:

- *Alcohol*: no storage capacity within the body and so all ingested alcohol is oxidized immediately. This response dominates oxidative pathways and reduces the rates at which other fuels are oxidized.

- *Protein*: limited storage capacity as body protein, which is accessible only through loss of lean body mass. Amino-acid metabolism is tightly regulated to ensure the oxidation of any excess.

- *Carbohydrate*: small capacity for storage as glycogen. The intake and oxidation of carbohydrate are very tightly "autoregulated", rapid and substantial changes in carbohydrate oxidation taking place in response to alterations in carbohydrate intake. Excess carbohydrate can also be converted into fat, but this metabolic pathway is not used by humans to any appreciable extent unless a large excess of a low-fat, high-carbohydrate diet is consumed. When carbohydrate is oxidized, however, less fatty-acid oxidation is required so that dietary fat is stored and endogenous fat retained. About 60–80% of the excess energy may be stored on carbohydrate overfeeding (*13*).

- *Fat*: the capacity for fat storage in the body is virtually unlimited and excess dietary fat does not markedly increase fat oxidation. Excess dietary fat is readily stored in adipose tissue depots with a very high efficiency (about 96%).

Thus, the bulk of the evidence suggests that carbohydrate and protein balances, but not fat balance, are well regulated. It is becoming clear that weight changes following challenges to body weight are due primarily to disruptions in fat balance, as these account for most of the imbalance produced in total energy (*13–19*).

In the long term, however, fat balance has to be regulated in order to achieve energy and macronutrient balance. Achieving fat balance again following a perturbation in energy balance is thought to require a change in the body fat mass. This may be because fat oxidation varies directly with body fat mass (20), but the way in which fat mass and total fat oxidation are linked is not clear. As an example, an increase in dietary fat without a rapid change in fat oxidation will produce a positive fat balance and hence lead to increases in body fat mass. As body fat mass increases, fat oxidation also increases. Fat mass will increase to the point at which fat oxidation matches fat intake, and the body fat mass will then stabilize at the new, higher, level.

Food palatability and pleasure. The palatability of food has an important influence on behaviour (3). Food palatability tends to promote consumption and is one of the most powerful influences in inducing a positive rather than a negative energy balance. It increases both the rate of eating and the sense of hunger during and between meals. The presence of fat in food is particularly enjoyable, and is associated with a pleasurable mouth-feel. The food industry has capitalized on this phenomenon by developing foods of increasing palatability. Moreover, the pleasurable sensations provided by foods can be viewed as a reward by those consuming them and can condition behaviour that favours overconsumption.

Sweetness is one of the most powerful, easily recognized and pleasurable tastes, so that many foods are sweetened in order to increase their palatability and consumption. The consumption of sugars does, however, lead to a subsequent suppression of energy intake by an amount roughly equivalent to the amount provided by the sugars (21). Nevertheless, sweetened foods of high fat content are expected to be conducive to excess energy consumption since palatability is enhanced both by sweetness and mouth-feel, and fat has only a small suppressive effect on appetite and intake. A preference for sweet–fat mixtures has been observed in obese women and may be a factor in promoting excess energy consumption (22).

Overview of macronutrient influence on body weight regulation. Table 7.2 summarizes the main characteristics of the macronutrients. Fat appears to be the key macronutrient that undermines the body's weight regulatory systems since it is very poorly regulated at the level of both consumption and oxidation. There is currently no consensus regarding the role of sugar intake on body weight regulation but there is some concern that the overconsumption of sweet–fat foods may be a

Table 7.2
Characteristics of macronutrients

Characteristic	Protein	Carbohydrate	Fat
Ability to bring eating to an end	High	Intermediate	Low
Ability to suppress hunger	High	High	Low
Contribution to daily energy intake	Low	High	High
Energy density	Low	Low	High
Storage capacity in body	Low	Low	High
Metabolic pathway to transfer excess intake to another compartment	Yes	Yes	No
Autoregulation (ability to stimulate own oxidation on intake)	Excellent	Excellent	Poor

problem, at least in certain subgroups of the population. Finally, although high protein intakes may appear to be advantageous in controlling energy intake and contributing to good body weight regulation, such intakes (especially of animal protein) have been associated with a number of adverse health consequences.

Dietary patterns

Daily eating pattern. Research on eating patterns and health has focused mainly on fluctuations in blood glucose and blood lipid concentrations throughout the day, particularly in the context of the control of NIDDM. There does appear to be some advantage in nibbling versus gorging under isocaloric conditions from the point of view of glycaemic control and hypertriglyceridaemia (23). However, in at least one controlled study, there was no effect of meal patterns on energy metabolism and energy balance (24).

Under free-living conditions, meal patterns vary widely across populations and cultures. Regular (high-fat) snacking has been associated with increased overall dietary intake in affluent societies, but this conclusion remains controversial (25). Other evidence from affluent societies suggests that dietary restraint and slimming leads to skipping breakfast and that this may result in overconsumption later in the day (26). Some people exhibit additional eating during the night, possibly as part of a night-eating syndrome (27) that is associated with obesity, although the mechanism underlying this association is not known. Recently, in a study in obese people trying to lose weight, it was found that the prognosis of weight loss was better in women who ate more and smaller meals than in those who ate fewer but larger meals.[1]

---

[1] Astrup A. ed. *Food and eating habits*, 1996. Background paper prepared by the Food and Eating Habits subgroup of the International Obesity Task Force.

Eating disorders. Eating disorders, particularly those that result in excess energy intake relative to requirements, have been implicated in the development of obesity. However, it is uncertain whether obesity is a direct result or an underlying cause of such disorders. For a more detailed discussion of eating disorders, including binge-eating disorder and night-eating disorder, see section 4.10.4.

7.3.2 *Physical activity patterns*

Cross-sectional data often reveal an inverse relationship between BMI and physical activity (*28–31*), indicating that obese and overweight subjects are less active than their lean counterparts. However, such correlations do not demonstrate cause and effect relationships, and it is difficult to be certain whether obese individuals are less active because of their obesity or whether a low level of activity caused the obesity. Results of other types of study, however, suggest that low and decreasing levels of activity are primarily responsible; for instance, obesity is absent among elite athletes while those athletes who give up sports frequently experience an increase in body weight and fatness (*32–35*). Furthermore, the secular trend in the increased prevalence of obesity seems to parallel a reduction in physical activity and a rise in sedentary behaviour. One of the best examples of this is provided by Prentice & Jebb (*36*), who used crude proxies for inactivity, such as the amount of time spent viewing television or the number of cars per household. These studies all suggest that decreased physical activity and/or increased sedentary behaviour plays an important role in weight gain and the development of obesity. This conclusion is further supported by prospective data. Dietz & Gortmaker (*37*), for example, have shown that the amount of television watching by young children is predictive of BMI some years later, while Rissanen et al. (*34*) have shown that a low level of physical activity during periods of leisure in adults is predictive of substantial weight gain (≥5 kg) in 5 years' time. More prospective data will help to clarify this relationship, but it seems reasonable to link physical inactivity with future weight gain.

Physical activity patterns have an important influence on the physiological regulation of body weight. In particular, they affect total energy expenditure, fat balance and food intakes. Box 7.1 outlines the different components of "physical activity" and defines "physical inactivity". Box 7.2 introduces the concept of physical activity levels (PALs).

Contribution of physical activity to total energy expenditure
Increased energy expenditure is an intrinsic feature of physical activity and exercise. Energy requirements increase from basal levels

Box 7.1

Physical activity

Physical activity is a global term referring to "any bodily movement produced by skeletal muscle that results in a substantial increase over the resting energy expenditure". It has three main components (*38*):

- *Occupational work*: activities undertaken during the course of work.

- *Household and other chores*: activities undertaken as part of day-to-day living.

- *Leisure-time physical activity*: activities undertaken in the individual's discretionary free time. Activity is selected on the basis of personal needs and interests. It includes exercise and sport:

  — *Exercise*: a planned and structured subset of leisure-time physical activity that is usually undertaken for the purpose of improving or maintaining physical fitness.

  — *Sport*: defined differently around the world but usually implies a form of physical activity that involves competition. It may also embrace general exercise and a specific occupation.

The time allocated to each of the three components varies considerably between individuals and populations.

Physical inactivity (sedentary behaviour)

Physical inactivity, or sedentary behaviour, can be defined as "a state when body movement is minimal and energy expenditure approximates RMR" (*39*). However:

- Physical inactivity represents more than an absence of activity; it also includes participation in physically passive behaviours such as television viewing, reading, working at a computer, talking with friends on the telephone, driving a car, meditating or eating (*40*).

- Physical inactivity may contribute to weight gain through means other than a reduction in energy expenditure. For example, recent studies in adolescents (*41*) and adults (*42*) have demonstrated significant relationships between inactivity and other adverse health practices, such as the consumption of less healthy foods and an increased fat intake.

immediately after the initiation of physical activity, and the increase persists for the duration of the activity. The total amount of energy expended depends on the characteristics of the physical activity (mode, intensity, duration and frequency) and of the individual performing the exercise (body size, level of habituation and fitness). These relationships have been extensively reviewed in the literature (*43*), and tables providing approximate values of the energy costs of various physical activities are widely available.

If exercise is vigorous, oxygen consumption remains elevated above resting levels for some time after exercise ceases. This metabolic response is called the "excess post-exercise oxygen consumption" (EPOC) and is due to the need to restore energy reserves, especially glycogen levels in liver and muscles. Compared with the energy cost of exercise itself, however, the contribution of EPOC is likely to be modest. In a recent study, it was estimated that, after 2 hours' exercising at a moderate intensity, it accounted for an extra 200 kJ/day

($48 kcal_{th}$/day) when averaged over 24 hours (*44*). Although this is quite small in terms of total daily energy expenditure, it has the potential to help maintain energy balance if exercise is undertaken regularly.

In addition to the immediate energy costs of increased physical activity and of the recovery period (i.e. EPOC), habitual exercise may influence several other components of energy expenditure including RMR. Although this area of research is still the subject of controversy, several recent studies have provided evidence for a positive association between activity levels and RMR (*45*). As the increase in the RMR is lost after several days of inactivity, this highlights the benefit of regular and sustained exercise patterns (*46*). Moreover, resistance exercise such as weight training may contribute to the maintenance of, or to an increase in, muscle mass, thereby favouring an elevation of the RMR or preventing a decrease in metabolic rate in the presence of weight loss (*47*).

Energy expenditure across the world
There is a widespread belief that daily life in less developed countries demands a much greater physical effort; for instance, a woman in a developing country spends 30–150 minutes every day of her life simply fetching water (*48*), and walks while attending to her daily chores for up to 1.5 hours. However, it is difficult to get accurate assessments of energy expenditure in free-living conditions; where developed and developing countries have been compared, few differences have been found (*49*). One explanation offered for this apparent discrepancy is that adults in less developed countries compensate by being inactive whenever possible; in Ethiopia, for example, energy expended on physical activity decreases in the post-harvest season (*50*). Secondly, the curtailment of physical activity in order to save energy represents the first line of defence against energy stress caused by insufficient dietary energy. Such a behavioural response can be illustrated by poorly nourished Rwandan women, who spend more time in low-cost activities than their better nourished counterparts (*51*). Overall, however, it is reasonable to conclude that people in less developed countries who spend a considerable portion of their time in finding food for their next meal and on personal chores are expending more energy in work and physical activity for a given body size than those in more developed countries.

Effect of physical activity on fat and substrate balance
Regular physical activity and substrate balance. One of the most important adaptations to regular exercise is the increased capacity to use fat

rather than carbohydrate during moderate physical activity. These differences become considerable when the exercise is maintained over a longer period; physically trained individuals metabolize more fat at given levels of energy expenditure than the untrained. It has been shown, for example, that the rate of fat oxidation in a group of unfit individuals increased by approximately 20% after a 12-week fitness training programme (52).

Of particular relevance is the observation that regular moderate physical exertion allows free-living volunteers to consume *ad libitum* a 40% fat diet without storing excess fat, whereas the same individuals, when sedentary, are in positive fat and energy balance and thus have a greater risk of becoming overweight and obese with time. If, however, they are offered a 20% fat diet, they remain in balance even when sedentary (53). Although these physiological studies should be interpreted with caution, they are of profound significance because they suggest a fundamental interaction between the level of physical activity and the proportion of dietary fat in determining whether energy balance can be sustained. The precise level of dietary fat that overwhelms the body's capacity to increase fat oxidation in response to increases in exercise and the extent to which this dietary fat level varies between individuals are unknown. However, it is thought that people who sustain moderate or high levels of physical activity throughout life can tolerate diets with a high fat content (e.g. 35–40% of energy) whereas lower fat intakes (20–25% of energy) may be needed to minimize energy imbalance and weight gain in sedentary individuals and societies. Thus, since most people in developed countries are sedentary, it is reasonable to assume that fat balance is achieved at a level of fat intake of 30% or less. In developing countries, the level of dietary fat compatible with fat balance may be higher as a result of the amount of energy expended on work and personal chores.

Exercise intensity and substrate balance. The metabolic responses to low- and high-intensity physical activity are very different. The extent to which fat and carbohydrate contribute to energy metabolism depends on the intensity level of the activity; fat is preferentially oxidized during low-intensity activity whereas carbohydrate is the dominant fuel at high intensity. In theory, the highest relative level of fat oxidation occurs when adults are moderately active at around 50–60% of maximum. In addition, theoretical calculations suggest that multiple bouts of intense exertion are better stimuli for fat oxidation than the equivalent energy use through more prolonged low-activity levels (54). The important point to remember is that the number of grams of fat oxidized during activity increases with the intensity and the duration of the activity, despite the fact that the proportion of fat in the mixture of fuel oxidized for muscular contraction may decrease at higher intensities. It should also be kept in mind that fat is oxidized not only during the activity but also in the recovery period.

Impact of physical activity on food intake and preference

Food intake. There is a common perception that exercise stimulates appetite, leading to an increased food intake that even exceeds the energy cost of the preceding activities. In fact, there is little supporting evidence for this from human studies; if a compensatory rise in intake does occur, this tends to be accurately matched to expenditure in lean subjects so that energy balance is re-established in the long term (54, 55). However, Woo et al. (56) showed that obese women did not compensate for the higher energy expenditure induced by exercise by increased intake, and thereby obtained a significant negative energy balance on exercise. This suggests that those who have stored an excess amount of energy may particularly benefit from exercise.

In the short term, hunger can be suppressed by intense exercise, and possibly by low-intensity exercise of long duration (54). The effect is short-lived, however, so that the temporal aspects of exercise-induced anorexia may best be measured by the delay in eating rather than the amount of food consumed (57).

Food preference. Whether exercise influences the type of food and the mix of macronutrients chosen by free-living subjects remains uncertain. In a small number of longitudinal studies, a higher intake of carbohydrate-rich foods has been observed with an increase in PAL (58), and a significant positive relation was recently found between the level of PAL and carbohydrate intake in a diet intervention study (59). However, it is not known whether dietary advice on optimum sport nutrition or physiological needs helps to initiate such dietary changes (54).

More information is needed in order to assess the value of a higher intake of carbohydrate-rich foods in the general population in whom changes in the level of physical activity are relatively small.

Physical activity levels for prevention of excessive weight gain

Analyses of over 40 national physical activity studies worldwide show that there is a significant relationship between the average BMI of adult men and their PAL, the likelihood of becoming overweight being substantially reduced at PALs of 1.8 or above (see Box 7.2, p. 114, for information on PALs). The relationship for women, though not statistically significant, is similar, but their physical activity tends to be lower (mean PAL 1.6) (49). It has been suggested, therefore, that people should remain physically active throughout life and sustain a PAL of 1.75 or more in order to avoid excessive weight gain. Sedentary people living or working in cities typically have a PAL of only 1.55–1.60, and PALs in industrialized societies are drifting downwards.

People who make extensive and increasing use of motorized transport, automated work and sedentary leisure pursuits, may find it difficult to attain PAL levels at or above 1.75 simply by increasing activity during "leisure time". This is illustrated by the calculations of Ferro-Luzzi & Martino (49), who showed that, for an average 70-kg adult male, increasing a PAL of 1.58 to one of about 1.70 involves an average of 20 minutes a day of vigorous exercise, such as running or circuit training at an activity ratio of 11 (a level of activity achievable only by a physically fit person), or else 1 hour of extra walking every day. Increasing a PAL of 1.58 to one of 1.76 requires approximately 1 hour and 40 minutes of extra walking (at 4 km/h) per day (Fig. 7.4). As these activity requirements are *additional* to a 24-minute period of "active leisure" (12 minutes of sports and 12 minutes of walking) already required for a PAL of 1.58, it follows that urban sedentary populations are likely to attain a PAL of 1.75 or more only if supported by vigorous national policies that encourage physical activity. For example, these should encourage children to be active at play and school, and should create environments in which walking and cycling become the most common means of travel to work and for short journeys.

7.4 Environmental and societal influences

As previously mentioned, the rapid increase in obesity rates in recent years has occurred in too short a time for there to have been any significant genetic changes within populations. This suggests that the primary cause of this increase must be sought in the environmental and societal changes now affecting a large proportion of the world's population.

This section discusses the environmental and societal factors that, through their effects on food intake and physical activity patterns, have overwhelmed the physiological regulatory processes that operate to keep weight stable in the long term. The societal changes that influence food intake and physical activity are also briefly considered.

7.4.1 Changing societal structures

The trend towards industrialization and an economy based on trade within a global market in most of the developing countries has

Figure 7.4

Active leisure required to achieve an overall mean PAL of 1.76[a]

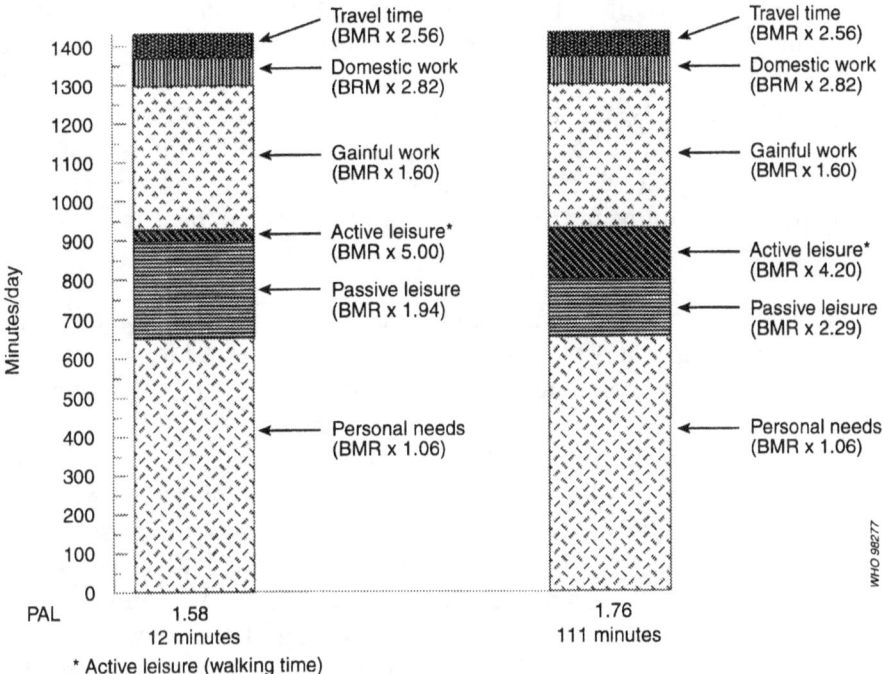

* Active leisure (walking time)

This model of the nature, duration and timing of active leisure required to achieve an overall mean PAL of 1.76 is based on the activity profile of the average Italian adult male, aged 30–60 years (60). He is assumed to weigh 70 kg and to have a predicted BMR of 1690 kcal$_{th}$/day. He is sedentary, being employed in a light-activity job (BMR factor = 1.60 (61)), and he spends only 24 minutes per day in active leisure (made up of 12 minutes' sports and 12 minutes' walking) at an overall BMR factor of 5.0. The other 252 minutes are spent in passive leisure (BMR factor 1.94). Increasing his daily walking time (speed 4 km/h, BMR factor 4.0) to 111 minutes raises his daily PAL to 1.76. The extra 99 minutes of walking time have been taken from the 252 minutes of passive leisure time; more specifically, it has been assumed that he would replace all the time spent watching television (90 minutes) and 9 minutes spent reading by walking.

[a] Adapted from reference 49 with the permission of the publisher. Copyright John Wiley & Sons Ltd.

brought about a number of improvements in the standard of living and in the services available to the population. However, it has also had various negative consequences; these have led, directly and indirectly, to deleterious nutritional and physical activity patterns that contribute to the development of obesity. Changing societal structures resulting from this economic transition have given rise to new problems associated with unemployment, overcrowding, and family and community breakdown. Social dislocation has often followed the loss by indigenous populations of traditional lands that are then used for production for the export market (62).

The food system that has emerged today is based on an industrial approach to agriculture and food production, makes most foods available regardless of season, and supplies highly processed outputs. While this may have contributed to improved food availability, it has not necessarily solved the problem of undernutrition in many of the poorer countries, nor has it improved the nutritional quality of the diets of the affluent (63). Indeed, some aspects of the industrialization of food production have contributed to the consumption of a diet higher in protein and fat (particularly saturated fat) and lower in complex carbohydrate.

The decline in energy expenditure seen with modernization and other societal changes is associated with a more sedentary lifestyle in which motorized transport, mechanized equipment, and labour-saving devices both in the home and at work have freed people from physically arduous tasks (Table 7.3). Work-related activity has declined over recent decades in industrialized countries, while leisure time dominated by television viewing and other physically inactive pastimes has increased (49). In the United Kingdom, for instance, the average distance walked by English children aged 14 years and younger fell by 20% between 1985 and 1992, and the average distance cycled fell by 26%, while the average distance travelled by car increased by 40% (64). The dangers of traffic and fears for personal safety have also influenced the decline of play in public areas.

Some of the key changes in societal structures that are thought to underlie the observed adverse changes in dietary and physical activity patterns implicated in the rapid global rise in obesity are considered below.

Modernization
Most adults who still have a "traditional" lifestyle appear to gain little or no weight with age. Anthropometric studies have reported an absence of obesity in the few remaining hunter–gatherer populations of the world, since energy expenditure is generally high and food supplies are scarce in certain periods of the year (70). For the majority of the world's population, however, the process of "modernization" has had a profound effect on the environment and on lifestyles over the last 50–60 years.

Food is now more abundant and the overall energy demand of modern life has dropped appreciably. These changes have subsequently been associated with dramatic increases in obesity rates. Indeed, Trowell & Burkitt, who carried out 15 case-studies of epidemiological

Table 7.3
Examples of energy-saving activity patterns in modern societies

Transport	Dramatic increases in car ownership mean that many people now travel short distances by car rather than walking or cycling to their destination.
In the home	Easily available fuel supplies obviate the need to collect and prepare fuels for lighting and heating; central heating has reduced the need to expend energy on thermoregulation. Energy expenditure is also reduced through the use of cooking equipment and ready-prepared foods/ingredients in meal preparation. Use of washing machines and vacuum cleaners makes for easier and quicker cleaning.
In the workplace	Mechanization, robotics, computerization and control systems have markedly reduced the need for even moderate activity, and only a very small proportion of the population now engages in physically demanding manual work.
Public places	Lifts, escalators and automatic doors are all designed to save substantial amounts of time and energy.
Sedentary pursuits	Television viewing is a major cause of inactivity, especially in the obese (65). Data from the USA show that it was strongly related to the incidence of new cases of obesity and to the failure of obese children to lose weight (37). These results are consistent with those of recent research showing that there were notable reductions in obesity when reductions in television viewing time were included in a dietary and activity intervention (66). The average person now watches over 26 hours of television a week in the United Kingdom, compared with 13 hours in the 1960s (67); children in the USA can spend more time watching television than attending school (68). Data are needed from other countries and for other sedentary pursuits such as computer use.
Urban residence	In urban areas of more affluent countries, children, women and older people are reluctant to go out alone or at night because of fears for their personal safety. Children also have difficulty in playing on streets in residential areas because of traffic trying to bypass congested main roads (69). For active leisure pursuits, children and adults therefore usually travel by car to sports facilities or to the open country as "special" outings rather than taking exercise routinely as a part of their daily lives. Further research is needed in this area to determine the relative importance of such factors, and whether or not they have an impact on obesity.

change in modernizing societies, report that obesity is the first of the so-called "diseases of civilization" to emerge (71). While early studies concluded that obesity usually emerged first in middle-aged women and then in middle-aged men, particularly among the more affluent groups, in the last decade it has become clear that obesity is increasingly being seen in much younger age groups, e.g. in children and adolescents. Trend or longitudinal data generally indicate that steady increases in the rates of obesity are greater in urban areas (72). However, a recent report from Samoa noted a dramatic increase in obesity prevalence of 297% in men and 115% in women in a rural community (73). This was clearly apparent even in the 25–34-year age group in both sexes.

New World syndrome. Obesity can be seen as the first wave of a defined cluster of NCDs now observed in both developed and developing countries. This has been called the "New World syndrome" (74) and is already creating an enormous socioeconomic and public health burden in poorer countries. High rates of obesity, NIDDM, hypertension, dyslipidaemia and CVD, coupled with cigarette smoking and alcohol abuse, are closely associated with the modernization/acculturation process and increasing affluence. The New World syndrome is responsible for disproportionately high levels of morbidity and mortality in newly industrialized countries, including eastern Europe, as well as among the ethnic minorities and the disadvantaged in developed countries (74). Thus, while obesity is viewed by health professionals from a medical perspective, it also needs to be recognized as a symptom of a much larger global social problem.

Economic restructuring and transition to market economies
The world is going through a period of rapid economic transition. Economies based on a few primary commodities are no longer viable, and a great deal of investment is often required to modernize existing industries and infrastructures in order to compete in a global market.

For many countries, the economic transition has meant huge loans from international banks as well as investments by large multinational companies on terms more favourable to them than to the host country. Interest payments on these loans coupled with rising interest rates have crippled health, education and social services, and local economies have been restructured to rely on industries based on cheap labour (63). Thus, many developing countries are becoming increasingly reliant on imported non-traditional foods, have very high rates of unemployment, and are also faced with the large-scale migration of people from rural to urban areas in search of work that is becoming increasingly sedentary in nature (75, 76).

Increasing urbanization

In less developed countries, urban residents are generally taller, heavier, and have a higher BMI than those who live in rural areas (72). This association between urban residence and obesity is of particular concern given the increasing numbers of people living in urban areas. Europe and North America are no longer the only major urban regions of the globe. Since the Second World War, the proportion of people living in the urban areas of less developed countries has increased from 16.7% in 1950 to 37% in 1994, and is predicted to grow to 57% in 2025 (77). Furthermore, there has been a shift towards the concentration of population growth in a few large cities of population greater than 5 million, often called urban agglomerations, and a shift in poverty to the urban areas, particularly into squatter and slum zones.

Urban residence is associated with a wide range of factors that in turn affect diet, physical activity and body composition. These include changes in transportation, access to and use of modern educational and health facilities, communications, marketing and availability of food, and large differences in occupational profiles, among others. In most countries, urban residents consume smaller proportions of carbohydrates and greater proportions of protein and fat, particularly saturated fat (78).

Changes in the role of women

In industrialized societies, an increasing number of women are entering the job market or are returning to full- or part-time paid employment within a few years of childbirth. They still tend to take responsibility for the health and well-being of the family but less and less for the more time- and energy-consuming domestic chores concerned with cleaning and the preparation and serving of food.

Going out to work has given women greater economic influence, especially over domestic purchases, and has contributed to the demand for convenience foods and labour-saving devices such as the microwave oven. People in paid employment tend to spend less time on shopping, cooking and other household tasks, so that the demand for "convenience" food products has increased. People may no longer have the time, energy, motivation or skills to prepare food from the basic ingredients. In the USA, the percentage of food dollars spent on eating outside the home increased by about 40% between 1980 and 1990 (79).

Changes in social structures

Changes in social structures have also led to an increasing proportion of the population working in service, clerical and other professional occupations that demand considerably less energy expenditure than the physically demanding manual work of more traditional societies.

Globalization of world markets
Food and food products are now commodities that are produced, traded and sold for profit in a market that is no longer largely local but increasingly global. Foods are less often seen as a matter of life and death, or of religious or cultural significance. Manufacturers and re-tailers seek to minimize uncertainties and costs, and to maximize returns. Competition is intense, both within and outside areas where these manufacturers and retailers are operating (*80*).

Large companies have expanded to control ever-increasing shares of trade in agriculture, manufacturing and retailing, and smaller farms and shops are being squeezed out of business (*81*). The effects of the debt crisis in the developing countries, the collapse of communism in eastern Europe and the former Soviet Union, and the dominance of free-market ideologies are promoting globalization and the develop-ment of market economies throughout the world, drawing even the most isolated self-supporting peasants into a global market (*63*). The concentration of food supply in the hands of a small number of multinational companies reduces their responsiveness to consumer or government pressure, and increases their influence on government policy (*82*).

7.4.2 *Variation within societies*

Socioeconomic status and obesity
Socioeconomic status is usually measured in terms of a composite index combining income, education, occupation and, in some devel-oping countries, place of residence (urban/rural). However, its indi-vidual components may have independent and even opposite effects on dietary intake and physical activity patterns, so that it is often very difficult to make generalizations about the relationship between socioeconomic status and obesity.

Despite these problems, studies have repeatedly shown that high socioeconomic status is negatively correlated with obesity in devel-oped countries, particularly among women, but positively correlated with it in populations of developing countries (*83, 84*). Further evi-dence suggests that, as the less developed countries attain higher levels of affluence, the positive relationship between socioeconomic status and obesity is slowly replaced by the negative correlation seen in developed countries (*78*).

Developing countries. In developing countries, the lower obesity rates observed in the populations of lower socioeconomic status are associated with a situation where people are limited in their ability to obtain enough food, yet still engage in moderate to heavy manual work and have little access to public transport. Hence, thin adults are considered poor, and overweight and obesity are a sign of affluence.

However, as per capita income increases, the nature of the diet in traditional societies tends to change in a pervasive and well documented manner (85). In particular, intakes of animal fat and protein increase, those of vegetable fat and protein decrease, those of total, and particularly complex, carbohydrates also decrease, and those of sugar increase.

The increase in income may be associated with increased away-from-home consumption of high-fat food items, as in the Philippines, or with increased consumption of meat, as in China. However, the overall effect tends to be a greater intake of total fat and an increased prevalence of obesity (78).

Developed countries. As previously mentioned, developed countries tend to show an inverse relationship between obesity and socioeconomic status, and between obesity and income, especially among women. A state of food deprivation is now very unusual in any major population groups in the industrialized countries, and the proportion of adults engaged in physical activity at home has fallen markedly with modernization. Thus, the groups of lower socioeconomic status need to be no more physically active or short of food (in energy terms) than those of higher status. In fact, studies suggest that families belonging to the lower-status groups engage in much less physical activity than those in higher ones; for instance, their obesity levels have risen in parallel with rising car ownership and they watch television for many more hours per day (36).

Studies indicate that change in income has little effect on dietary structure in countries where income levels are already quite high in relation to basic food needs; instead, increases in income are spent on more elaborately packaged and processed or higher-quality foods rather than on a greater quantity of food. In the poorest income groups, however, food demand is much more price- and income-sensitive, and many people struggle to obtain enough high-quality food for what is considered to be a healthy diet (86). The diet of households of lower socioeconomic status tends to be energy-dense, and high fat intakes are a prominent feature; the more expensive vegetables, fruit and whole-grain cereals are eaten more sparingly.

Education and health-related knowledge
Level of education appears to be inversely associated with body weight in industrialized countries. Surveys in France, the United

Kingdom and the USA all showed that the proportion of obese men and women was higher among those of a lower educational level (87, 88). The observed inverse relationship between education and body weight may be partly attributed to the fact that individuals of higher educational level are more likely to follow dietary recommendations and adopt other risk-avoidance behaviours than those of low educational attainment (89). In the USA, a trend has been emerging among the better educated sections of the population to adopt and adhere to dietary guidelines and other "healthy lifestyles" (78). Unfortunately, little is known about the relationship between education level and obesity in developing countries except that urban adults are more highly educated than those from rural areas.

The benefit of nutritional knowledge *per se* appears to be limited. Surveys indicate that, although some people know what constitutes a healthy diet, they prefer in practice to consume a relatively unhealthy one (90). Obesity rates continue to climb, despite the increased frequency of dieting among obese people, suggesting that knowledge and frequent attempts to slim are insufficient for successful weight control.[1] However, without these widespread attempts to control body weight, the prevalence of obesity in industrialized countries might be much higher.

7.4.3 *Cultural influences*

It is also essential in any international review of obesity to recognize that at least two-thirds of the world's population consists of people of African, Chinese or Indian origin, living in developing countries. For such people, the risk factors and perceived causes of obesity often differ from those of people of European origin.

Culture affects both food intake and physical activity patterns, although the "cultural attributes" responsible are not well characterized and accurately measured at present. Cultural behaviours and beliefs are learned in childhood, are often deeply held, and are seldom questioned by adults, who pass them on to their offspring. Attitudes and beliefs may change over time, however, as shown by the expectations in industrialized countries of body weight and shape that appear to be of particular importance in determining people's behaviour. Substantial differences in obesity prevalence between relatively affluent populations indicate that cultural values and traditions may mediate or moderate the effects of affluence on obesity rates.

---

[1] Westenhoefer J. In: *Social and cultural issues of obesity*, 1996. Background paper prepared by Social and Cultural subgroup of the International Obesity Task Force.

Cultural influences on food intake, selection and preparation
Cultural factors are among the strongest determinants of food choice. They include peer group pressures, social conventions, religious practices, the status assigned to different foods, the influence of other members of the household and individual lifestyles. The effect of cultural factors can be seen, for example, in children who give way to peer pressure by selecting high-fat foods, and in executives dining at expensive restaurants with business colleagues.

Cultural explanations of obesity are based on what are traditionally thought of as "learned" behaviours. For example, it is not uncommon for white American parents to encourage their children to eat particular foods by rewarding them with other food items. Recent research has shown that this culturally sanctioned pattern of rewards actually contributes to a dislike of the "good" foods and a preference for the "bad" ones (*91*). In some cultures, high-fat meals are provided for family entertainment and celebration.

Few foods are unique to particular cuisines, although some may be considered suitable for consumption by one culture but not by another. Human beings value food for much more than its nutrient content, and it is used to express relationships between people as well as in celebrating religious festivities, weddings and other important social occasions.

Attitudes towards health, fitness and activity. The idea of engaging in physical activity during leisure time is not understood in many cultures and communities in which energy conservation has historically been a prime concern especially during periods of food shortage. The improvement in food availability has done little to change such attitudes to physical activity, which often persist across generations even though the original rationale for their adoption has long been forgotten.

In contrast, the people of the Nordic countries, among others, prize fitness and vitality, and thus have a positive attitude towards physical activity; in such countries, considerable amounts of leisure time are devoted to vigorous activity rather than to more sedentary pursuits.

Body image. Throughout most of human history, increased weight and girth have been viewed as signs of health and prosperity. This is still the case in many cultures, especially where conditions make it easy to remain lean or where thinness in babies is associated with increased risk of infectious disease. Fat women are often viewed as attractive in Africa, for example, where some traditional communities have "fattening huts" for elite pubescent girls to ensure that they start their reproductive lives with a peripheral fat energy surplus (*84*). In Puerto Rican communities, weight gain after marriage is seen as showing that the husband is a good provider and that the woman is a good wife, cook and mother. Weight loss is socially discouraged, and there is a widespread fatalistic acceptance of the view that successful weight loss by the obese is not possible (*92*).

In many industrialized countries, the past three decades have witnessed a marked change in attitudes towards body shape and weight. Thinness in women has come to symbolize competence, success, control and sexual attractiveness, while obesity represents laziness, self-indulgence and a lack of will power.[1] Such ideals of thinness exist in a setting where it is easy to become fat, and tend to lead to inappropriate dieting, a failure to achieve unrealistic weight goals, and weight cycling. Recent research suggests that, as many traditional cultures embrace the values and ideals of the politically or economically dominant culture of the industrialized countries, they too are likely to see an increase in eating disorders and unhealthy weight-control practices (*93, 94*). In the USA, concern about overweight is seen in a variety of ethnic groups (*95*), although the preferred "unhealthy" method of weight control tends to vary; as compared with white adolescent females, Hispanics reported greater use of diuretics, Asians reported more binge eating, and African Americans reported higher rates of vomiting (*96*).

Cross-cultural research reveals that the male body ideal is most often related to "bigness" (large structure and muscularity), but not necessarily to fatness (*70, 97*). In contrast to women, men generally do not see increased size and adiposity as a problem, although they are at greater risk of developing abdominal obesity; they therefore tend not to seek the treatment they need.[2]

Television and popular magazines have been criticized for reinforcing the association between thinness and attractiveness (*98, 99*), especially when they present conflicting messages in the form of advertisements for energy-dense and high-fat foods. Media exposure and the presentation of thin female fashion models as the ideal increase many women's dissatisfaction with their body shape and promote eating disorders (*100, 101*). Efforts should be made to ensure that the media do not create a situation in which obesity is stigmatized and eating

---

[1] Hill AJ. In: *Social and cultural issues of obesity*, 1996. Background paper prepared by Social and Cultural subgroup of the International Obesity Task Force.
[2] Astrup A, ed. *Food and eating habits*, 1996. Background paper prepared by Food and Eating Habits subgroup of the International Obesity Task Force.

disorders promoted in the many societies where such a situation does not exist.

7.4.4 *Impact of societal changes on food intake and activity patterns*

Governments, the food industry, the media and consumers, among others, have the potential to influence, positively and negatively, the impact of societal and environmental factors, particularly modernization, on the food supply and on PALs. None of them in isolation has been responsible for creating an obesity-promoting environment any more than, acting alone, any one of them can effect meaningful change. Thus a partnership is clearly required if such an environment is to be avoided.

Governments and regional authorities

Governments and regional authorities are responsible for protecting and promoting the health of the community by ensuring access to a safe, nutritious and affordable food supply as well as to facilities for regular physical activity. Modernization and the competing demands of economic development and health have sometimes created a situation where actions by governments have contributed to a decrease in physical activity and an increase in the intake of energy-dense food, contrary to their own health guidelines.

Development and adaptation of national dietary guidelines. Dietary recommendations and guidelines have often not kept pace with societal changes and advances in nutrition science or with the specific nutritional problems of communities as countries go through the nutrition transition.

Government nutrition programmes. Government feeding programmes established in developing countries to deal with undernutrition often remain in place even when there is evidence to suggest that undernutrition no longer exists. Such programmes may sometimes contribute to a worsening of the problem of overconsumption of energy that follows modernization.

Meals provided in government institutions. Governments and regional authorities are responsible for the food served in schools, hospitals, day-care centres and government organizations. Even when they do not provide such food, they have the power to lay down firm guidelines as to its quality and composition. Unfortunately, many have failed to draw up guidelines for the provision of meals in such establishments and to monitor their implementation.

Physical activity at school. Governments and regional authorities are in a position to ensure that regular physical activity is undertaken in all schools. However, many have allowed the time devoted to such activity in schools to be reduced and land on which children previously played in safety to be used for other purposes.

Regulation of food quality, advertising and labelling. Many governments have failed to respond to the changing food supply by laying down or amending food regulations governing food quality and safety, and the labelling and advertising of foods. This has led to a situation in which consumers are at risk of being badly informed or confused by poor labelling or the unregulated marketing of foods. A recent report by Consumers International (*102*) has shown that, even when regulations governing marketing and advertising exist, they are often not enforced so that compliance with them is poor.

Food production policies. Economic development and increasing involvement in free markets often result in the abandonment by governments of a food production policy based on small regional food producers and the adoption instead of one that involves large-scale or centralized farming. Such policies often increase the movement of people from rural areas to towns and cities and can result in a loss of food diversity and of the production of traditional foodstuffs in favour of the wide-scale production of cash crops for export markets.

The aim in many developing countries is still that of increasing the total food energy available to the population so that the problems of undernutrition are avoided. However, the increased emphasis in food production on oil crops or meat products may add to the problems associated with the rapidly increasing energy density of the national diet, especially when these products make their way into the local food supply and displace traditional foods that are no longer widely available.

Food surpluses. For many decades, the primary objective of governments and the food industry has been to maintain a supply of cheap food so that even the poorest sections of society can purchase sufficient amounts. The use of tax concessions, direct subsidies and rebates from the producer to the retailer, however, have often led to an oversupply of commodities, so that economic strategies now tend to be directed at increasing consumer demand to meet supply. As a result, surplus cheaper foodstuffs are exported from developed countries to markets created in developing ones (*103*). This is illustrated by the export of cheap vegetable fats from Australia, the USA and

Europe to neighbouring countries in the Pacific, South America, Asia and eastern Europe (*76, 104*).

The food industry

Advances in food technology and product development. Technological advances in cultivating, preserving, producing, transporting and storing foods have increased the year-round availability of a wider variety of foods to a larger number of people. The continuing globalization of these processes means that such trends in food availability are spreading from industrialized countries to developing ones.

Advances in food technology have also contributed to the consumption of diets increasingly dependent on processed foods. It is now possible to produce food products having almost any variety of taste, textural quality and nutrient content. In fact, food characteristics are often manipulated to such an extent that it is difficult for individuals to associate visual, textural or taste cues with the energy content of meals. This is especially important given the increasing trend towards prepackaged foods and the concomitant decline in the use of natural and basic ingredients in food preparation in the home.[1] Consumers are losing control over the preparation of the foods that they eat, and food composition is increasingly being placed in the hands of manufacturers.

In order to survive in the modern competitive market economies, businesses cannot stand still but need to grow and maintain or increase profits for shareholders. If this cannot be done by increasing sales of basic foodstuffs to those who can afford to buy them, it can be done by turning basic foodstuffs into other, more expensive products (i.e. processed, prepackaged foods) (*63*).

Fast foods. Although it can be argued that "fast foods" have been available for centuries, such foods tended to be those of traditional diet and culture. Today, fast foods and snacks tend to be universal in nature, are often provided by large multinational corporations, and are high in fat, low in complex carbohydrates, and energy-dense (*105*). They may not be entirely satisfying and are often used as regular additions to the diet instead of being consumed as an occasional meal or treat.[2] Furthermore, beverages containing substantial amounts of sugar or alcohol are often consumed as part of a fast-food meal.

---

[1] Buisson DH. *Consumer food choices for the 2000s — the impact of social and marketing trends.* Paper presented at the CSIRO Food Industry Conference, Adelaide, Australia, 1992.

[2] Astrup A, ed. *Food and eating habits*, 1996. Background paper prepared by Food and Eating Habits subgroup of the International Obesity Task Force.

Modern fast foods have proliferated rapidly, and are widely available and intensively advertised. In 1991, it was reported that fast foods accounted for 19% of the global consumer catering market, then worth US$ 730 000 million, and that their market share was expected to grow to 25% by 2000. In the USA, the market for fast foods was worth US$ 78 000 million in 1992 (*106*), and more than 200 people are served a hamburger every second of the day. Greater availability has been achieved by increasing the number of outlets and the opportunities to eat outside the home; the number of fast-food outlets in the United Kingdom doubled in the 10 years between 1984 and 1993, while the number of restaurants and cafes remained the same (*107*).

Direct evidence that increased consumption of fast foods leads to overweight and obesity is lacking. However, it is widely perceived that this is the case and that obesity has increased in industrialized societies as families turn away from home-prepared meals and consume more fast or take-away foods. The roles of the media and of the consumer in this process are considered below.

Marketing and advertising. The commercialization of food manufacturing and retail outlets has encouraged enthusiastic marketing. Larger portion sizes give the consumer an impression of "better value" for money, and marketing strategies such as "eat all you can for X dollars" represent an encouragement to eat beyond natural biological limits. Furthermore, these foods and outlets are backed by substantial advertising campaigns that, in stark contrast to public health or nutrition campaigns, are extremely persuasive and successful.[1]

The media
The media, including television, radio and print, play a major role in disseminating information in modern consumer societies. They are part of informal education, and both reflect and influence public attitudes. However, far more money has been spent on promoting high-fat/energy-dense foods than on promoting healthier foods. For example, £86.2 million was spent on promoting chocolate confectionery in the United Kingdom in 1992 compared with only £4 million spent on advertising fresh fruit, vegetables and nuts (*108*).

The media provide information on new and existing foods to consumers and have a pervasive influence on food choice; they have clearly been influential in changing dietary patterns in recent decades.

---

[1] Astrup A, ed. *Food and eating habits*, 1996. Background paper prepared by Food and Eating Habits subgroup of the International Obesity Task Force.

Television, in particular, plays a major role in informing and influencing children. This development may not be helpful, e.g. 91% of foods advertised during peak children's viewing time in the USA, and a similar proportion in the United Kingdom, were high in fat, sugar and/or salt (*109, 110*). Although the food and advertising industries consistently argue that food advertising has little influence or detrimental effect on children's eating habits, a considerable amount of evidence now suggests that it does influence food selection by children and adolescents, especially among susceptible groups (*63, 111*). Television viewing appears closely linked to the consumption by children of the foods that they see advertised on television (*112, 113*).

Consumers
Consumers play a role in fuelling a demand for a wide variety of products and services conducive to weight gain; they often demand processed and convenience meals that tend to be high in fat and energy-dense, as well as labour-saving devices both at home and in the workplace that require little energy expenditure. Although it is recognized that consumer demand is itself influenced by a number of factors, including marketing, advertising, culture, fashion and convenience, the product or service is unlikely to survive in its existing form if consumers do not want it. Better educated consumers can demand better products, especially those of improved nutritional quality.

Most societies have a preference for sweet foods and prize fatty foods the most (*114*). With increasing incomes and the greater availability of such foods, there has been a marked increase in their consumption. The ability to purchase labour-saving devices is widely welcomed by consumers in all societies and ownership of a car is seen as an important status symbol. Consumers in emerging economies are likely to be reluctant to return to diets of traditional foods, to physical labour or to walking, all of which are associated with poverty, once a certain level of income has been achieved.

7.5 Individual/biological susceptibility

Epidemiological, genetic and molecular studies of populations all over the world suggest that some people are more susceptible than others to becoming overweight and obese, and that such susceptible individuals exist in countries differing widely in lifestyle and environmental conditions.

Obesity is commonly seen as a complex multifactorial disease; it is a condition resulting from a lifestyle that promotes a positive energy balance, but also one that becomes manifest more readily in people who have an inherited susceptibility to be in positive energy balance.

Furthermore, no two obese individuals are the same; there are differences in both the degree and the regional distribution of excess body fat as well as in the fat topography response of individuals to factors that promote weight gain. Such differences are due not only to genetic variation but also to the prior experiences and environments to which the individuals have been exposed. The evidence for this conclusion has been carefully reviewed (*115*). However, considerable uncertainty remains as to the genes and mutations involved, and how they operate and interact to enhance the susceptibility of some individuals to obesity.

The evidence for a role of genetic, biological and other factors in determining the susceptibility of individuals to weight gain and obesity is briefly discussed here.

7.5.1 *Genetic susceptibility*

The role of genetic factors in weight gain is currently the subject of much research, and the discovery of leptin (see pp. 136–137) has led to a renewed interest in genetic and metabolic influences in the development of obesity. While it is possible that single or multiple gene effects may cause overweight and obesity directly, and indeed do so in some individuals, this does not appear to be the case in the majority of people. Instead, it is currently considered that the genes involved in weight gain increase the risk or susceptibility of an individual to the development of obesity when exposed to an adverse environment. Only in the case of certain genetic disorders are particular gene effects "necessary" for obesity expression.

Heritability
The level of heritability is the fraction of population variation in a trait (e.g. BMI) that can be explained by genetic transmission, and a large number of twin, adoption and family studies on the heritability of different measures of obesity have been conducted. Adoption studies tend to generate the lowest estimates and twin studies the highest. Recently, however, the application of complex analytical techniques to databases encompassing all three types of studies has led to the conclusion that the true heritability of BMI in large sample sizes was likely to be in the range 25–40% (*116, 117*). On the other hand, similar genetic epidemiological research has shown that the profile of fat distribution was also characterized by a significant heritability level of the order of about 50% of the total human variation. Finally, recent studies have shown that the amount of abdominal fat was influenced by a genetic component accounting for 50–60% of the individual differences (*118, 119*).

Obesity tends to run in families, obese children frequently having obese parents. However, there is a dearth of data concerning the level of risk of developing obesity for a first-degree relative of an overweight, moderately obese or severely obese person in comparison with the population prevalence of the condition (*117*). One of the first papers on this topic by Allison et al. (*120*) concluded that the relative risk was about 2 for overweight, increasing to about 3–4 for higher levels of obesity.

Gene–environment interactions

While some individuals are prone to excessive accumulation of fat and struggle to lose weight, others do not have these difficulties. Studies in both animals and humans suggest that genetic factors are partially responsible for such differences in the tendency of individuals to gain fat when chronically exposed to a positive energy balance.

For example, by feeding a high-fat diet to different inbred strains of mice, scientists have found that both sensitive and resistant strains exist (*121*). More recently, a prospective study showed that high fat intake in humans was correlated with subsequent weight gain only in those subjects who were overweight at baseline and had obese parents (*122*). These studies and others suggest that the genetic predisposition to obesity observed in animal models may also exist in humans, making some individuals particularly susceptible to a high fat intake.

It is also quite clear that certain inbred strains of rodents are particularly prone to becoming obese when exposed to overfeeding or to a highly palatable diet. Similarly, in a study on pairs of identical twins, the body weight and the proportion of fat gained in response to controlled overfeeding was significantly more alike within pairs of twins than between them (*123*). This and other studies based on the same design strongly suggest that there are individuals who are more likely than others to gain body mass and body fat when challenged by an energy overload. Thus, the responsiveness to energy intake and dietary composition is partly dependent on specific genetic factors that have yet to be clearly identified.

Types of genetic effects

If the heritability estimates are correct — and the evidence for this is quite strong — the genes are exerting their influence on body mass and body fat as a result of DNA sequence variation either in the coding sequence of the genes or in the segments that affect gene expression. It is obvious that most of the genes contributing to obesity do not qualify as necessary genes, i.e. genes that cause obesity whenever one or two copies of the defective allele are present. Indeed, the genetic susceptibility seems to be rather one caused by genes associated with an increase in the proneness to gain weight over time or, alternatively, by the absence of genetic influences that protect against the development of a positive energy balance. In general, such genes exert smaller effects on the phenotype than necessary genes—a situation that makes the identification of these genes and of the responsible mutations much more difficult. Nonetheless, even though the genetic effect associated with the risk of obesity appears to be of the multigenic type, there is some indirect evidence to support the notion that one or a few genes may play a more important role. In other words, obesity is a truly complex multifactorial phenotype with a genetic component that includes both polygenic and major gene effects.

A series of studies reported over the past several years strongly supports the view that many genes are involved in causing susceptibility to obesity. Several types of research have been used to identify these genes and the specific DNA sequence variation responsible for the increase in risk of becoming obese. The evidence accumulated so far has recently been reviewed (124) and provides statistical or experimental support for a role for about 70 genes, loci or markers. Many more years of research will be needed before the important genes and critical mutations are finally identified for both excess body fat content and upper body and abdominal fat accumulation.

Possible mechanisms whereby genetic susceptibility may operate include:

- *Low RMR*: e.g. studies in the Pima Indians have shown RMR clusters in families and that those with lower RMR have a greater risk of gaining 10 kg in the following 5 years (125, 126).

- *Low rate of lipid oxidation*: e.g. a low ratio of fat to carbohydrate oxidation under standardized conditions is a risk factor for subsequent weight gain (18, 127).

- *Low fat-free mass*: a low fat-free mass for a given body mass is a risk factor for subsequent weight gain as it tends to depress the level of RMR, thus favouring a positive energy balance.

- *Poor appetite control*: e.g. if satiety is reached at a high level of energy intake, the net result is likely to be a positive energy balance and weight gain. Here, many genes and molecules are currently under investigation. For instance, leptin, the hormone product of the *ob* or leptin gene, is an important satiety factor secreted by the adipose tissue in humans. An anomaly in the leptin receptor gene may be associated with leptin resistance in humans. However, the

Table 7.4
Some factors involved in the development of obesity thought to be genetically modulated

Macronutrient-related:
  adipose tissue lipolysis
  adipose tissue and muscle lipoprotein lipase (LPL) activity
  muscle composition and oxidative potential
  free fatty acids and β-receptor activities in adipose tissue
  capacities for fat and carbohydrate oxidation (respiratory quotient)
  dietary fat preferences
  appetite regulation
Energy expenditure:
  metabolic rate
  thermogenic response to food
  pattern of energy usage (nutrient partitioning)
  propensity for spontaneous physical activity
Hormonal:
  insulin sensitivity
  growth hormone status
  leptin action

genetic mutations that result in leptin insufficiency and lead to obesity in mice are not thought to exist in humans.

Many other factors, some of which are listed in Table 7.4, are currently under intensive investigation.

The place of genetic research on obesity
While research aimed at identifying genes for use in screening, and ultimately in therapy, is important, it will be many years before the results can be applied in practice. At present, the greatest value of genetic research on obesity is in the increased understanding of the pathophysiology of the disease that it provides.

7.5.2 *Non-genetic biological susceptibility*

In addition to the genetic influences discussed in section 7.5.1, a number of other biological factors have been shown to influence an individual's susceptibility to weight gain and the development of obesity. These are discussed below.

Sex
A number of physiological processes are believed to contribute to an increased storage of fat in females. Such fat deposits are believed to be essential in ensuring female reproductive capacity. Studies in humans and animals indicate that females exhibit a stronger preference

for carbohydrate before puberty while males prefer protein. However, after puberty, both males and females display a marked increase in appetite for fat in response to changes in the gonadal steroid levels. This rise in fat appetite occurs much earlier and to a greater extent in females (*128*).

Females have a tendency to channel extra energy into fat storage while males use more of this energy for protein synthesis. This pattern of energy usage, or "nutrient partitioning", in females contributes to further positive energy balance and fat deposition for two reasons. First, the storage of fat is far more energy-efficient than that of protein, and second, it will lead to a lowering of the lean-to-fat tissue ratio with the result that RMR does not increase at the same rate as body mass.

Ethnicity

Ethnic groups in many industrialized countries appear to be especially susceptible to the development of obesity and its complications. Evidence suggests that this may be due to a genetic predisposition to obesity that only becomes apparent when such groups are exposed to a more affluent lifestyle. This is demonstrated graphically by the following:

- *Pima Indians of Arizona*: members of this tribe, which has a very high prevalence of obesity (*129*), gained weight after abandoning their traditional lifestyle.

- *Australian Aboriginals*: this ethnic group tends to have a high incidence of central adiposity, hypertension and NIDDM, but this can be reduced or eliminated within a very short period simply by reverting to a more traditional lifestyle (*130*, *131*). Similar reductions in obesity and cardiovascular risk have been observed when natives in Hawaii have returned to a traditional diet after abandoning the usual modern diet (*132*).

- *South Asians overseas*: the prevalence of NIDDM and mortality from CHD are higher in people of south Asian (Bangladeshi, Indian and Pakistani) descent living in urban societies than in other ethnic groups. This is related to a greater tendency to accumulate intra-abdominal fat for a given BMI compared with other populations (*133*).

It appears from the foregoing that a number of ethnic groups are more prone to the risks of obesity when exposed to the lifestyle common in industrialized countries. For the majority, this problem seems to result from a combination of genetic predisposition and a change from the traditional to a more affluent and sedentary lifestyle and its accompanying diet. However, susceptibilities to obesity comorbidities are not uniform across groups. In Mexico, for example, NIDDM is more common than hypertension among the obese population, whereas in other areas of the world CVD may be more common.

Other environmental factors may also be important in promoting obesity in ethnic minority groups in industrialized countries, e.g. in African Americans in the USA, where the highest rates of obesity are found in the poorest communities. In these populations, fat-rich, energy-dense diets are likely to be the cheapest, and reduced levels of activity stem from unemployment. Other factors associated with poverty may also be involved.

The problem of obesity in ethnic minorities demonstrates the need for targeted prevention and intervention strategies.

Critical periods for weight gain
Although a general rise in body weight and a modest increase in percentage body fat over the lifespan can be expected in developed countries, at least until 60–65 years of age (*134*), recent studies have shown the importance of nutrition during certain critical periods when an individual may be more vulnerable to the development of obesity in the future. However, until longitudinal studies have been completed, the contribution of each of the periods shown in Table 7.5 to the prevalence of obesity and its comorbidities remains unclear (*135*).

7.5.3 *Other factors promoting weight gain*
An individual's tendency to gain weight may be increased by certain factors such as smoking cessation, the development of a disease, or treatment with drugs that promote weight gain as a side-effect. These are considered briefly below.

Smoking cessation
Smoking causes a marked increase in metabolic rate and tends to reduce food intake compared with that of non-smokers (*2*). It may also cause a longer-term increase in RMR, although the evidence for this is conflicting (*148, 149*).

Smoking and body weight are inversely related (*150*), and smokers frequently gain weight when they give up the habit. Williamson (*151*) studied a nationally representative cohort of smokers and non-smokers in the USA (1971–1984) and found that the mean weight gain attributable to smoking cessation was 2.8 kg in men and 3.8 kg in

Table 7.5
Critical periods for the development of obesity

Critical period	Reason for increased risk
Prenatal	Nutrition during fetal life may contribute directly to the development of the size, shape and composition of the body, and to the metabolic competence to handle macronutrients. Close relationships exist between patterns of intrauterine growth and the risk of abdominal fatness, obesity and their comorbidities in later life (136–138).
Adiposity rebound (5–7 years)	BMI begins to increase rapidly after a period of reduced adiposity during the preschool years. This period coincides with increased autonomy and socialization and so may represent a stage when the child is particularly vulnerable to the adoption of behaviours that both influence and predispose to the development of obesity. It is uncertain whether early adiposity rebound is associated with an increased risk of persistent obesity in later life (139–141).
Adolescence	A period of increased autonomy often associated with irregular meals, changed food habits and periods of inactivity during leisure combined with physiological changes that promote increased fat deposition, particularly in females (142, 143).
Early adulthood	Early adulthood is usually a period of marked reduction in physical activity. In women, this usually occurs between the ages of 15 and 19 years but in men it may be as late as the early 30s (144).
Pregnancy	It has been claimed that a mother's BMI increases with successive pregnancies. However, recent evidence suggests that this increase is likely to be on average less than 1 kg per pregnancy, although the range may be wide and is associated with total weight gained during pregnancy (145). Many study designs confound changes in weight with ageing and changes in weight with parity (146). In many developing countries, consecutive pregnancies at short intervals are often associated with weight loss rather than with weight gain.
Menopause	In industrialized societies, weight generally increases with age but it is not clear why menopausal women are particularly prone to rapid weight gain. The loss of the menstrual cycle does affect food intake and reduces metabolic rate slightly, although most of the weight gain has been attributed to reduced activity (147).

women. However, heavy smokers (more than 15 cigarettes per day) and younger people were at higher risk of major weight gain (>13 kg) after giving up smoking.

Notwithstanding the risk of gaining weight, it is important to understand that smoking cessation should be a higher priority than weight

Table 7.6
Drugs that may promote weight gain

Drug	Main condition treated or other use
Tricyclic antidepressants, lithium	Depression
Sulfonylureas	NIDDM
β-Adrenergic blockers	Hypertension
Some steroid contraceptives	Contraception
Corticosteroids	Various diseases
Insulin	NIDDM
Cyproheptadine	Allergy, hay fever
Valproic acid, neuroleptics	Epilepsy
Phenothiazine	Psychosis
Pizotifen	Migraine headache

loss in obese patients who smoke; a large number of prospective studies have shown that smoking has a larger impact on morbidity and mortality than any small rise in BMI (*152–156*). The beneficial effects of giving up smoking are unlikely to be negated by the weight gain that may follow.

Excess alcohol intake
As previously mentioned, the body is unable to store alcohol, and oxidation of ingested alcohol is given priority over that of other macronutrients. Alcohol consumption therefore meets some of the body's energy needs, allows a greater proportion of energy from other foods eaten to be stored,[1] and is thus associated with an increased risk of abdominal fat (*155*). However, in epidemiological studies, those with the greatest alcohol intakes tend to be thinner (*156, 157*), perhaps because such people eat less and have a large part of their energy requirements met by alcohol (*158*).

Drug treatment
The use of the drugs listed in Table 7.6 can promote weight gain. Adults on long-term corticosteroid therapy for rheumatoid arthritis may be at particular risk of weight gain, since the side-effects of the drug exacerbate the effects of limited physical activity.

Disease states
Certain genetic disorders, as well as some endocrinological conditions such as hypothyroidism, Cushing disease and hypothalamic tumours,

---

[1] Astrup A, ed. *Food and eating habits*, 1996. Background paper prepared by Food and Eating Habits subgroup of the International Obesity Task Force.

can cause weight gain. However, these are extremely rare causes of obesity, accounting for only a very small proportion of obesity in the population.

Major reduction in activity
In some individuals, a major reduction in activity without a compensatory decrease in habitual energy intake may be the major cause of increased adiposity. Examples include the weight gain often observed in elite athletes when they retire, in young people who sustain sports injuries, in young people in wheelchairs after accidents or in others who develop arthritis.

Changes in social and environmental circumstances
Marriage (159), the birth of a child, a new job and climate change can all lead to undesirable changes in eating patterns and consequent weight gain.

7.6 Weight loss

Although many people are successful in losing weight, between a half and one-third of this weight loss is commonly regained over the following year (160). This weight regain is independent of the extent of the initial weight loss or the techniques used to assist weight loss. The first year after losing weight is considered to be a particularly difficult period for weight regain prevention, because biological and behavioural processes act to drive body weight back to baseline levels (144). Despite the difficulty of achieving and maintaining weight loss over long periods, some people succeed in doing so (161). Study of these individuals may provide some clues that will help to explain their success.

References

1. Cummings JH et al. A new look at dietary carbohydrate: chemistry, physiology and health. *European Journal of Clinical Nutrition*, 1997, 51:417–423.

2. Dallosso HM, James WPT. The role of smoking in the regulation of energy balance. *International Journal of Obesity*, 1984, 8:365–375.

3. Blundell JE, King NA. Overconsumption as a cause of weight gain: behavioural–physiological interactions in the control of food intake (appetite). In: Chadwick DJ, Cardew GC, eds. *The origins and consequences of obesity*. Chichester, Wiley, 1996:138–158 (Ciba Foundation Symposium 201).

4. Schutz Y. Macronutrients and energy balance in obesity. *Metabolism*, 1995, 44(9 Suppl. 3):7–11.

5. Diaz EO et al. Metabolic response to experimental overfeeding in lean and overweight healthy volunteers. *American Journal of Clinical Nutrition*, 1992, 56:641–655.

6. Klein S, Goran M. Energy metabolism in response to overfeeding in young adult men. *Metabolism: Clinical and Experimental*, 1993, 42:1201–1205.

7. Leibel RL, Rosenbaum M, Hirsch J. Changes in energy expenditure resulting from altered body weight. *New England Journal of Medicine*, 1995, 332:621–628.

8. Porikos KP, Hesser MF, van Itallie TB. Caloric regulation in normal weight men maintained on a palatable diet of conventional foods. *Physiology and Behavior*, 1982, 29:293–300.

9. Lissner L, Heitmann BL. Dietary fat and obesity: evidence from epidemiology. *European Journal of Clinical Nutrition*, 1995, 49:79–90.

10. Popkin BM et al. Dietary and environmental correlates of obesity in a population study in China. *Obesity Research*, 1995, 3(Suppl. 2):135s–143s.

11. Tordoff MG, Reed DR. Sham feeding sucrose or corn oil stimulates food intake in rats. *Appetite*, 1991, 17:97–103.

12. Raben A, Macdonald I, Astrup A. Replacement of dietary fat by sucrose or starch: effects on 14 days ad libitum energy intake, energy expenditure and body weight in formerly obese and never-obese subjects. *International Journal of Obesity and Related Metabolic Disorders*, 1997, 21:846–859.

13. Horton TJ et al. Fat and carbohydrate overfeeding in humans: different effects on energy storage. *American Journal of Clinical Nutrition*, 1995, 62:19–29.

14. Flatt JP et al. Effects of dietary fat on postprandial substrate oxidation and on carbohydrate and fat balances. *Journal of Clinical Investigation*, 1985, 76:1019–1024.

15. Acheson KJ et al. Glycogen storage capacity and de novo lipogenesis during massive carbohydrate overfeeding in man. *American Journal of Clinical Nutrition*, 1988, 48:240–247.

16. Flatt JP. Importance of nutrient balance in body weight regulation. *Diabetes/Metabolism Reviews*, 1988, 4:571–581.

17. Schutz Y, Flatt JP, Jéquier E. Failure of dietary fat intake to promote fat oxidation: a factor favouring the development of obesity. *American Journal of Clinical Nutrition*, 1989, 50:307–314.

18. Zurlo F et al. Low ratio of fat to carbohydrate oxidation as predictor of weight gain: study of 24-hour RQ. *American Journal of Physiology*, 1990, 259:E650–E657.

19. Bennett C et al. The short-term effects of dietary fat ingestion on energy expenditure and nutrient balance. *American Journal of Clinical Nutrition*, 1992, 55:1071–1077.

20. Astrup A et al. Obesity as an adaptation to a high-fat diet: evidence from a cross-sectional study. *American Journal of Clinical Nutrition*, 1994, 59:350–355.

21. **Anderson GH.** Sugars, sweetness and food intake. *American Journal of Clinical Nutrition*, 1995, 62(1 Suppl.):195S–201S.

22. **Drenowski A.** Human preference for sugar and fat. In: Fernstrom JD, Miller GD, eds. *Appetite and body weight regulation: sugar, fat and macronutrient substitutes*. Boca Raton, FL, CRC Press, 1994:137–147.

23. **Jenkins DJ et al.** Nibbling versus gorging: metabolic advantages of increased meal frequency. *New England Journal of Medicine*, 1989, 321:929–934.

24. **Verboeket-van de Venne WP, Westerterp KR, Vester AD.** Effect of the pattern of food intake on human energy metabolism. *British Journal of Nutrition*, 1993, 70:103–115.

25. **Drummond S, Crombie N, Kirk T.** A critique of the effects of snacking on body weight status. *European Journal of Clinical Nutrition*, 1996, 50:779–783.

26. **Holt S et al.** Relationship of satiety to postprandial glycaemic, insulin and cholecystokinin responses. *Appetite*, 1992, 18:129–141.

27. **Stunkard A et al.** Binge eating disorder and the night-eating syndrome. *International Journal of Obesity and Related Metabolic Disorders*, 1996, 20:1–6.

28. **Rising R et al.** Determinants of total daily energy expenditure: variability in physical activity. *American Journal of Clinical Nutrition*, 1994, 59:800–804.

29. **Schulz LO, Schoeller DA.** A compilation of total daily energy expenditures and body weights in healthy adults. *American Journal of Clinical Nutrition*, 1994, 60:676–681.

30. **Davies PS, Gregory J, White A.** Physical activity and body fatness in pre-school children. *International Journal of Obesity and Related Metabolic Disorders*, 1995, 19:6–10.

31. **Westerterp KR, Goran MI.** Relationship between physical activity related energy expenditure and body composition: a gender difference. *International Journal of Obesity and Related Metabolic Disorders*, 1997, 21:184–188.

32. **Williamson DF.** Dietary intake and physical activity as "predictors" of weight gain in observational, prospective studies of adults. *Nutrition Reviews*, 1996, 54(4 Pt 2):S101–S109.

33. **Haapanen N et al.** Association between leisure time physical activity and 10-year body mass change among working-aged men and women. *International Journal of Obesity and Related Metabolic Disorders*, 1997, 21:288–296.

34. **Rissanen AM et al.** Determinants of weight gain and overweight in adult Finns. *European Journal of Clinical Nutrition*, 1991, 45:419–430.

35. **Williamson DF et al.** Recreational physical activity and ten-year weight change in a US national cohort. *International Journal of Obesity and Related Metabolic Disorders*, 1993, 17:279–286.

36. **Prentice AM, Jebb SA.** Obesity in Britain: gluttony or sloth? *British Medical Journal*, 1995, 311:437–439.

37. **Dietz WH, Gortmaker SL.** Do we fatten our children at the television set? Obesity and television viewing in children and adolescents. *Pediatrics*, 1985, **75**:807–812.

38. **Bouchard C, Shephard RJ.** Physical activity, fitness and health: the model and key concepts. In: Bouchard C et al., eds. *Physical activity, fitness and health: international proceedings and consensus statement.* Champaign, IL, Human Kinetic Publishers, 1994.

39. **Dietz WH.** The role of lifestyle in health: the epidemiology and consequences of inactivity. *Proceedings of the Nutrition Society*, 1996, **55**:829–840.

40. **Ainsworth BE et al.** Compendium of physical activities: classification of energy costs of human physical activities. *Medicine and Science in Sports and Exercise*, 1993, **25**:71–80.

41. **Lytle LA et al.** Covariance of adolescent health behaviours: the class of 1989 study. *Health Education Research*, 1995, **10**:133–146.

42. **Simoes EJ et al.** The association between leisure-time physical activity and dietary fat in American adults. *American Journal of Public Health*, 1995, **85**:240–244.

43. **Hill JO et al.** Physical activity and energy requirements. *American Journal of Clinical Nutrition*, 1995, **62**(5 Suppl.):1059S–1066S.

44. **Goldberg GR et al.** Residual effect of graded levels of exercise on metabolic rate. *European Journal of Clinical Nutrition*, 1990, **44**:99–105.

45. **Westerterp KR et al.** Body mass, body composition and sleeping metabolic rate before, during and after endurance training. *European Journal of Applied Physiology and Occupational Physiology*, 1994, **69**:203–208.

46. **Tremblay A et al.** Effect of a three-day interruption of exercise-training on resting metabolic rate and glucose-induced thermogenesis in training individuals. *International Journal of Obesity*, 1988, **12**:163–168.

47. **Ballor DL et al.** Resistance weight training during caloric restriction enhances lean body weight maintenance. *American Journal of Clinical Nutrition*, 1988, **47**:19–25.

48. *The world's women 1970–1990: trends and statistics.* New York, United Nations, 1991.

49. **Ferro-Luzzi A, Martino L.** Obesity and physical activity. In: Chadwick DJ, Cardew GC, eds. *The origins and consequences of obesity.* Chichester, Wiley, 1996:207–227 (Ciba Foundation Symposium 201).

50. **Ferro-Luzzi A et al.** Seasonal energy deficiency in Ethiopian rural women. *European Journal of Clinical Nutrition*, 1990, **44**(Suppl. 1):7–18.

51. **Shetty PS, James WPT.** Functional consequences of low BMI in adults. In: *Body mass index. A measure of chronic energy deficiency in adults.* Rome, Food and Agriculture Organization of the United Nations, 1994 (FAO Food and Nutrition Paper Series, No. 56).

52. **Hurley BF et al.** Muscle triglyceride utilization during exercise: effect of training. *Journal of Applied Physiology*, 1986, **60**:562–567.

53. **Stubbs RJ et al.** Covert manipulation of the ratio of dietary fat to carbohydrate and energy density: effect on food intake and energy balance in free-living men eating ad libitum. *American Journal of Clinical Nutrition*, 1995, **62**:330–337.

54. **Saris WHM.** Physical activity and body weight regulation. In: Bouchard C, Bray GA, eds. *Regulation of body weight. Biological and behavioural mechanisms.* Chichester, Wiley, 1996:135–147.

55. **Woo R, Pi-Sunyer FX.** Effect of increased physical activity on voluntary intake in lean women. *Metabolism: Clinical and Experimental*, 1985, **34**:836–841.

56. **Woo R, Garrow JS, Pi-Sunyer FX.** Effect of exercise on spontaneous caloric intake in obesity. *American Journal of Clinical Nutrition*, 1982, **36**:470–477.

57. **King NA, Burley VJ, Blundell JE.** Exercise-induced suppression of appetite: effects on food intake and implications for energy balance. *European Journal of Clinical Nutrition*, 1994, **48**:715–724.

58. **Janssen GME, Graef CJJ, Saris WHM.** Food intake and body composition in novice athletes during a training period to run a marathon. *International Journal of Sports Medicine*, 1989, **10**(Suppl. 1):S17–S21.

59. **Westerterp KR, Verboeket-van de Venne WPHG, Bouten CVC.** Energy expenditure and physical activity in subjects consuming full or reduced fat products as part of their normal diet. *British Journal of Nutrition*, 1996, **96**:785–795.

60. *Indagine multiscopo sulle famiglie, Anni 1987–1991. No 4 L'uso del tempo in Italia. [Multi-purpose household survey, 1987–1991. No. 4 Time use in Italy.]* Rome, Instituto di Statistica, 1993.

61. *Energy and protein requirements. Report of a Joint FAO/WHO/UNU Expert Consultation.* Geneva, World Health Organization, 1985 (WHO Technical Report Series, No. 724).

62. **McMichael PD.** *Development and social change: a global perspective.* Thousand Oaks, CA, Pine Forge Press, 1996.

63. **Tansey G, Worsley T.** *The food system. A guide.* London, Earthscan, 1995.

64. **DiGuiseppi C, Roberts I, Li L.** Influence of changing travel patterns on child death rates from injury: trend analysis. *British Medical Journal*, 1997, **314**:710–713.

65. **Buchowski MS, Sun M.** Energy expenditure, television viewing and obesity. *International Journal of Obesity and Related Metabolic Disorders*, 1996, **20**:236–244.

66. **Epstein LE et al.** Effects of decreasing sedentary behaviour and increasing activity on weight change in obese children. *Health Psychology*, 1995, **14**:109–115.

67. **Office of Population Censuses and Surveys.** *General household survey.* London, Her Majesty's Stationery Office, 1994.

68. **Dietz WH, Strasburger VC.** Children, adolescents and television. *Current Problems in Pediatrics*, 1991, **21**:8–31.

69. James WP. A public health approach to the problem of obesity. *International Journal of Obesity and Related Metabolic Disorders*, 1995, **19**(Suppl. 3):S37–S45.

70. Brown PJ. Culture and the evolution of obesity. *Human Nature*, 1991, **2**:31–57.

71. Trowell HC, Burkitt DP. *Western diseases: their emergence and prevention*. Cambridge, MA, Harvard University Press, 1981.

72. Monteiro CA et al. The nutrition transition in Brazil. *European Journal of Clinical Nutrition*, 1995, **49**:105–113.

73. Hodge AM et al. Dramatic increase in the prevalence of obesity in Western Samoa over the 13 year period 1978–1991. *International Journal of Obesity and Related Metabolic Disorders*, 1994, **18**:419–428.

74. Gracey M. New World syndrome in Western Australian aborigines. *Clinical and Experimental Pharmacology and Physiology*, 1995, **22**:220–225.

75. Raikes P. *Modernising hunger: famine, food surplus and farm policy in the EEC and Africa*. London, Catholic Institute for International Relations/James Currey, 1988.

76. Drenowski A, Popkin BM. The nutrition transition: trends in the global diet. *Nutrition Reviews*, 1997, **55**:31–43.

77. *World urbanization prospects: the 1994 revisions*. New York, United Nations, 1995.

78. Popkin BM et al. A review of dietary and environmental correlates of obesity with emphasis on developing countries. *Obesity Research*, 1995, **3**(Suppl. 2):145S–153S.

79. Kinsey JD. Food and families' socioeconomic status. *Journal of Nutrition*, 1994, **124**(9 Suppl.):1878S–1885S.

80. Lang T, Hines C. *The new protectionism: protecting the future against free trade*. London, Earthscan, 1993.

81. Lang T. The public health impact of globalisation of food trade. In: Shetty PS, McPherson K, eds. *Diet, nutrition and chronic disease: lessons from contrasting worlds. Proceedings of the Sixth London School of Hygiene and Tropical Medicine Public Health Forum*. Chichester, Wiley, 1997:173–187.

82. McMichael AJ. The public health impact of globalisation of food trade: discussion. In: Shetty PS, McPherson K, eds. *Diet, nutrition and chronic disease: lessons from contrasting worlds. Proceedings of the Sixth London School of Hygiene and Tropical Medicine Public Health Forum*. Chichester, Wiley, 1997:187–193.

83. Sobal J, Stunkard AJ. Socioeconomic status and obesity; a review of the literature. *Psychological Bulletin*, 1989, **105**:260–275.

84. Brown P, Bentley-Condit VK. Culture, evolution and obesity. In: Bray GA, Bouchard C, James WPT, eds. *Handbook of obesity*. New York, Marcel Dekker, 1998:143–155.

85. *Provisional indicative world plan for agricultural development, Vol. 2*. Rome, Food and Agriculture Organization of the United Nations, 1970:500–505.

86. **Leather S.** *The making of modern malnutrition. An overview of food poverty in the UK.* London, The Caroline Walker Trust, 1996.

87. **Kuczmarski RJ.** Prevalence of overweight and weight gain in the United States. *American Journal of Clinical Nutrition*, 1992, **55**(2 Suppl.):495S–502S.

88. **Laurier D et al.** Prevalence of obesity: a comparative survey in France, the United Kingdom and the United States. *International Journal of Obesity and Related Metabolic Disorders*, 1992, **16**:565–572.

89. **Hulshof KF et al.** Diet and other life-style factors in high and low socio-economic groups (Dutch Nutrition Surveillance System). *European Journal of Clinical Nutrition*, 1991, **45**:441–450.

90. **Leitzmann C.** Ernährungsgewohnheiten von Oecotrophologiestudenten. [Food and nutrition behaviour of students of home economics and nutrition.] *Ernährungs-Umschau*, 1979, **26**:181–185.

91. **Birch LL.** Obesity and eating disorders: a developmental perspective. *Bulletin of the Psychonomic Society*, 1991, **29**:265–272.

92. **Massara EB.** *Que gordita! A study of weight among women in a Puerto Rican community.* New York, AMS Press, 1989.

93. **Craig PL, Caterson ID.** Body size, age, ethnicity, attitudes and weight loss. In: Ailhaud G et al., eds. *Obesity in Europe.* London, John Libbey, 1991:421–426.

94. **Craig PL et al.** Do Polynesians still believe that big is beautiful? Comparison of body size perceptions and preferences of Cook Islands, Maori and Australians. *New Zealand Medical Journal*, 1996, **109**:200–203.

95. **Snow JT, Harris MB.** Disordered eating in South-western Pueblo Indians and Hispanics. *Journal of Adolescence*, 1989, **12**:329–336.

96. **Story M et al.** Ethnic/racial and socioeconomic differences in dieting behaviors and body image perceptions in adolescents. *International Journal of Eating Disorders*, 1995, **18**:173–179.

97. **Cassidy CM.** The good body: when big is better. *Medical Anthropology*, 1991, **13**:181–213.

98. **Silverstein B et al.** The role of the mass media in promoting a thin standard of bodily attractiveness for women. *Sex Roles*, 1986, **14**:519–532.

99. **Nemeroff CJ et al.** From the Cleavers to the Clintons: role choices and body orientation as reflected in magazine article content. *International Journal of Eating Disorders*, 1994, **16**:167–176.

100. **Hamilton K, Waller G.** Media influences on body size estimation in anorexia and bulimia. An experimental study. *British Journal of Psychiatry*, 1993, **162**:837–840.

101. **Stice E et al.** Relation of media exposure to eating disorder symptomatology: an examination of mediating mechanisms. *Journal of Abnormal Psychology*, 1994, **103**:836–840.

102. *A spoonful of sugar. Television food advertising aimed at children: An international comparative survey.* London, Consumers International, 1996.

103. **Goodman D, Redclift M.** *Refashioning nature. Food, ecology and culture.* London, Routledge, 1991.

104. **Morgan N.** World vegetable oil consumption expands and diversifies. *Food Review*, 1993, **16**:26–30.

105. Massachusetts Medical Society, Committee on Nutrition. Fast food fare: consumer guidelines. *New England Journal of Medicine*, 1990, **321**:752–755.

106. *Fast food: the international market.* London, Euromonitor Market Direction, 1993.

107. *UK food market*, 4th ed. Hampton, England, Key Note, 1994.

108. *The food pocket book.* Henley-on-Thames, England, NTC Publications, 1994.

109. *Easy to swallow, hard to stomach.* London, National Food Alliance, 1995.

110. **Taras HL, Gage M.** Advertised foods on children's television. *Archives of Pediatrics and Adolescent Medicine*, 1995, **149**:649–652.

111. **Ray JW, Klesges RC.** Influences on the eating behavior of children. *Annals of the New York Academy of Sciences*, 1993, **699**:57–69.

112. **Taras HL et al.** Television's influence on children's diet and physical activity. *Journal of Developmental and Behavioral Pediatrics*, 1989, **10**:176–180.

113. **Robinson TN, Killin JD.** Ethnic and gender differences in the relationships between television viewing and obesity, physical activity, and dietary fat intake. *Journal of Health Education*, 1995, **26**(Suppl.):91–98.

114. **Fischler C.** *L'Homnivore: le goût, la cuisine et le corps.* [*The omnivore: taste, cooking and the human body.*] Paris, Odile Jacob, 1990.

115. **Bouchard C.** Genetics of obesity: overview and research directions. In: Bouchard C, ed. *The genetics of obesity.* Boca Raton, FL, CRC Press, 1994:223–233.

116. **Bouchard C.** Genetic influences on body weight and shape. In: Brownell KD, Fairburn CG, eds. *Eating disorders and obesity: a comprehensive handbook.* New York, Guilford Press, 1995.

117. **Bouchard C.** Genetics of obesity in humans: current issues. In: Chadwick DJ, Cardew GC, eds. *The origins and consequences of obesity.* Chichester, Wiley, 1996:108–117 (Ciba Foundation Symposium 201).

118. **Pérusse L et al.** Familial aggregation of abdominal visceral fat level — results from the Quebec family study. *Metabolism: Clinical and Experimental*, 1996, **45**:378–382.

119. **Bouchard C et al.** The genetics of human obesity. In: Bray GA, Bouchard C, James WPT, eds. *Handbook of obesity.* New York, Marcel Dekker, 1998:157–190.

120. **Allison DB, Faith MS, Nathan JS.** Risch's lambda values for human obesity. *International Journal of Obesity and Related Metabolic Disorders*, 1996, **20**:990–999.

121. **West DB et al.** Dietary obesity in nine inbred mouse strains. *American Journal of Physiology*, 1992, **262**(6 Pt 2):R1025–R1032.

122. **Heitmann BL et al.** Dietary fat intake and weight gain in women genetically predisposed for obesity. *American Journal of Clinical Nutrition*, 1995, **61**:1213–1217.

123. **Bouchard C et al.** The response to long-term overfeeding in identical twins. *New England Journal of Medicine*, 1990, **322**:1477–1482.

124. **Pérusse L et al.** The human obesity gene map: the 1996 update. *Obesity Research*, 1997, **5**:49–61.

125. **Bogardus C et al.** Familial dependence of the resting metabolic rate. *New England Journal of Medicine*, 1986, **315**:96–100.

126. **Ravussin E et al.** Reduced rate of energy expenditure as a risk factor for body-weight gain. *New England Journal of Medicine*, 1988, **318**:467–472.

127. **Eckel RH.** Insulin resistance: an adaptation for weight maintenance. *Lancet*, 1992, **340**:1452–1453.

128. **Leibowitz, SF.** Neurochemical–neuroendrocrine systems in the brain controlling macronutrient intake and metabolism. *Trends in Neurosciences*, 1992, **15**:491–497.

129. **Carter J et al.** Tribal differences in diabetes: prevalence among American Indians in New Mexico. *Public Health Reports*, 1989, **104**:665–669.

130. **O'Dea K, White NG, Sinclair AJ.** An investigation of nutrition-related risk factors in an isolated Aboriginal community in northern Australia: advantages of a traditionally-oriented life-style. *Medical Journal of Australia*, 1988, **148**:177–180.

131. **O'Dea K.** Westernization, insulin resistance and diabetes in Australian aborigines. *Medical Journal of Australia*, 1991, **155**:258–264.

132. **Shintani TT et al.** Obesity and cardiovascular risk intervention through the ad libitum feeding of traditional Hawaiian diet. *American Journal of Clinical Nutrition*, 1991, **53**(6 Suppl.):1647S–1651S.

133. **McKeigue PM.** Metabolic consequences of obesity and body fat pattern: lessons from migrant studies. In: Chadwick DJ, Cardew GC, eds. *The origins and consequences of obesity*. Chichester, Wiley, 1996:54–67 (Ciba Foundation Symposium 201).

134. **Rolland-Cachera MF et al.** Body mass index variations — centiles from birth to 87 years. *European Journal of Clinical Nutrition*, 1991, **45**:13–21.

135. **Dietz WH.** Critical periods in childhood for the development of obesity. *American Journal of Clinical Nutrition*, 1994, **59**:955–959.

136. **Ravelli GP, Stein ZA, Susser MW.** Obesity in young men after famine exposure in utero and early infancy. *New England Journal of Medicine*, 1976, **295**:349–353.

137. **Law CM et al.** Early growth and abdominal fatness in adult life. *Journal of Epidemiology and Community Health*, 1992, **46**:184–186.

138. **Jackson AA, Langley-Evans SC, McCarthy HD.** Nutritional influences in early life upon obesity and body proportions. In: Chadwick DJ, Cardew

GC, eds. *The origins and consequences of obesity.* Chichester, Wiley, 1996:118–137 (Ciba Foundation Symposium 201).

139. **Rolland-Cachera MF et al.** Adiposity rebound in children: a simple indicator for predicting obesity. *American Journal of Clinical Nutrition,* 1984, **39**:129–135.

140. **Siervogel RM et al.** Patterns of change in weight/stature from 2 to 18 years: findings from long-term serial data for children in the Fels longitudinal growth study. *International Journal of Obesity,* 1991, **15**:479–485.

141. **Prokopec M, Bellisle F.** Adiposity in Czech children followed from 1 month of age to adulthood: analysis of individual BMI patterns. *Annals of Human Biology,* 1993, **20**:517–525.

142. **Braddon FEM et al.** Onset of obesity in a 36 year birth cohort. *British Medical Journal Clinical Research Edition,* 1986, **293**:299–303.

143. **Must A et al.** Long-term morbidity and mortality of overweight adolescents. A follow-up of the Harvard Growth Study of 1922 to 1935. *New England Journal of Medicine,* 1992, **327**:1350–1355.

144. **Wing RR.** Changing diet and exercise behaviors in individuals at risk of weight gain. *Obesity Research,* 1995, 3(Suppl. 2):277S–282S.

145. **Ohlin A, Rössner S.** Maternal body weight development after pregnancy. *International Journal of Obesity,* 1990, **14**:159–173.

146. **Williamson DF et al.** A prospective study of childbearing and 10-year weight gain in US white women 25 to 40 years of age. *International Journal of Obesity and Related Metabolic Disorders,* 1994, **18**:561–569.

147. **Wing RR et al.** Weight gain at the time of menopause. *Archives of Internal Medicine,* 1991, **151**:97–102.

148. **Hofstetter A et al.** Increased 24-hour energy expenditure in cigarette smokers. *New England Journal of Medicine,* 1986, **314**:79–82.

149. **Warwick PM, Edmundson HM, Thomson ES.** No evidence for a chronic effect of smoking on energy expenditure. *International Journal of Obesity and Related Metabolic Disorders,* 1995, **19**:198–201.

150. **Grunberg NE.** Behavioral and biological factors in the relationship between tobacco use and body weight. In: Katkin ES, Manuck SB, eds. *Advances in behavioral medicine. Vol 2.* Greenwich, CT, JAI Press, 1986:97–129.

151. **Williamson DF.** Smoking cessation and severity of weight gain in a national cohort. *New England Journal of Medicine,* 1991, **324**:739–745.

152. **Willett WC et al.** Relative and absolute excess risks of coronary heart disease among women who smoke cigarettes. *New England Journal of Medicine,* 1987, **317**:1303–1309.

153. **Wannamethee G, Shaper AG.** Body weight and mortality in middle aged British men: impact of smoking. *British Medical Journal,* 1989, **299**:1497–1502.

154. **Fitzgerald AP, Jarrett RJ.** Body weight and coronary heart disease mortality: an analysis in relation to age and smoking habit: 15 years follow-

up data from the Whitehall study. *International Journal of Obesity and Related Metabolic Disorders*, 1992, **16**:119–123.

155. **Troisi RJ et al.** Cigarette smoking, dietary intake, and physical activity: effects on body fat distribution — the Normative Aging Study. *American Journal of Clinical Nutrition*, 1991, **53**:1104–1111.

156. **Gruchow HW et al.** Alcohol consumption, nutrient intake and relative body weight among US adults. *American Journal of Clinical Nutrition*, 1985, **42**:289–295.

157. **Colditz GA et al.** Alcohol intake in relation to diet and obesity in women and men. *American Journal of Clinical Nutrition*, 1991, **54**:49–55.

158. **Prentice AM.** Alcohol and obesity. *International Journal of Obesity and Related Metabolic Disorders*, 1995, **19**(Suppl. 5):S44–S50.

159. **Rauschenbach B, Sobal J, Frongillo EA Jr.** The influence of change in marital status on weight change over one year. *Obesity Research*, 1995, **3**(4):319–327.

160. **Wadden TA.** Treatment of obesity by moderate and severe caloric restriction. Results of clinical research trials. *Annals of Internal Medicine*, 1993, **119**:688–693.

161. **Klem ML et al.** A descriptive study of individuals successful at long-term weight maintenance of substantial weight loss. *American Journal of Clinical Nutrition*, 1997, **66**:239–246.

Addressing the problem of overweight and obesity

8. Principles of prevention and management of overweight and obesity

8.1 Introduction

Although there is still much to be learned about the complex and diverse factors involved in the etiology of weight gain and obesity, it is now clear that powerful societal and environmental forces influence energy intake and expenditure, and may overwhelm the physiological regulatory mechanisms that operate to keep weight stable. The susceptibility of individuals to these forces is affected by genetic and other biological factors, such as sex, age and hormonal activity, over which they have little or no control. Dietary factors and physical activity patterns are considered to be the major modifiable factors underlying excessive weight gain that, if corrected, can serve to prevent obesity.

The effective prevention and management of obesity should therefore focus on:

— elements of the social, cultural, political, physical and structural environment that affect the weight status of the community or population at large;
— processes and programmes to deal with those individuals and groups who are at particularly high risk of obesity and its comorbidities;
— management protocols for those individuals with existing obesity.

It is also important to recognize that, in many societies, an undue emphasis on thinness has been accompanied by an increased prevalence of eating disorders such as anorexia nervosa and bulimia. Interventions aimed at obesity prevention or management should therefore be carefully designed to avoid precipitating the development of eating disorders associated with undue fear of fatness, especially in young adolescent girls. Such interventions should also discourage other unhealthy behaviours, e.g. cigarette smoking, that may be adopted in the belief that they will prevent weight gain.

This section is concerned with the principles underlying prevention and management strategies for overweight and obesity, the different levels of preventive action, and the need to deal with individuals with existing obesity. It highlights the need for coordinated action in a variety of settings and shared responsibility on the part of key stakeholders. It is emphasized that:

• Coherent and comprehensive strategies for the effective prevention and management of obesity should focus on:

— elements of the environment that affect the weight status of the community or population at large;
— individuals and groups who are at particularly high risk of obesity and its comorbidities;
— management protocols for those individuals with existing obesity.

- Obesity management encompasses the following four key strategies:

  — prevention of weight gain;
  — promotion of weight maintenance;
  — management of obesity comorbidities;
  — promotion of weight loss.

- Indirect evidence from a variety of sources indicates that obesity is preventable and that the prevention of weight gain is easier, less expensive and more effective than treating obesity after it has fully developed. However, only limited research has been done in this area.

- Obesity prevention is not simply a matter of preventing individuals of normal weight from becoming obese. It also involves the prevention of overweight in such individuals, obesity in those who are already overweight, and weight regain in those who have been overweight or obese in the past but who have since lost weight.

- The traditional classification of disease prevention can be confusing when applied to a complex, multifactorial condition such as obesity, and can usefully be replaced by the following three levels (see also section 8.3.3):

  — universal/public health prevention (directed at everyone in a community);
  — selective prevention (directed at high-risk individuals and groups);
  — targeted prevention (directed at those with existing weight problems and those at high risk of diseases associated with overweight).

- A preliminary analysis of obesity management approaches adopted by existing national health care services in a range of countries has revealed wide variation between countries, and indicated that very few have a coherent and comprehensive range of services capable of providing the level of care required to manage obese patients effectively.

- The attitudes of health professionals towards obesity and its management are often negative, and knowledge and skills in managing obesity are seldom adequate. Training opportunities for family doctors and other health professionals are extremely limited in most countries.

- National commitment to obesity control should be a shared responsibility — consumers, governments, food industry/trade, and the media all have important roles to play in promoting effective changes in diet and everyday levels of physical activity. In national food and nutrition policies and public health policies obesity management and prevention should form part of NCD control programmes.

8.2 Strategies for addressing the problem of overweight and obesity

Until recently, obesity prevention and obesity management were perceived as two distinct processes, the former being aimed at preventing weight gain and the latter concerned with weight loss. Management was seen as the role of the clinician, whereas prevention was considered to be the domain of health promotion or public health departments. However, it is now realized that obesity management covers a whole range of long-term strategies ranging from prevention, through weight maintenance and the management of obesity comorbidities, to weight loss (1; see Fig. 8.1). The individual strategies are interdependent, so that truly effective obesity management must address all of them in a coordinated manner and in a variety of settings.

Strategies to deal with the immediate and existing health problems of those who are already obese often take precedence in discussions on obesity management. However, as Fig. 8.1 shows, considerably more attention needs to be given to prevention activities than is the case at present, as these are likely to have a much greater impact on the effective long-term control of obesity.

8.3 Prevention strategies

There are a number of reasons why strategies aimed at the prevention of weight gain and obesity should be easier, less expensive and potentially more effective than those aimed at treating obesity after it has fully developed:

- Obesity develops over time and, once it has developed, is difficult to treat. Indeed, a number of studies have shown that many obesity treatments fail to achieve long-term success (2–10).

- The health consequences of obesity are the result of the cumulative metabolic and physical stress of excess weight over a long period and may not be fully reversible by weight loss (11, 12).

Figure 8.1
Obesity management[a]

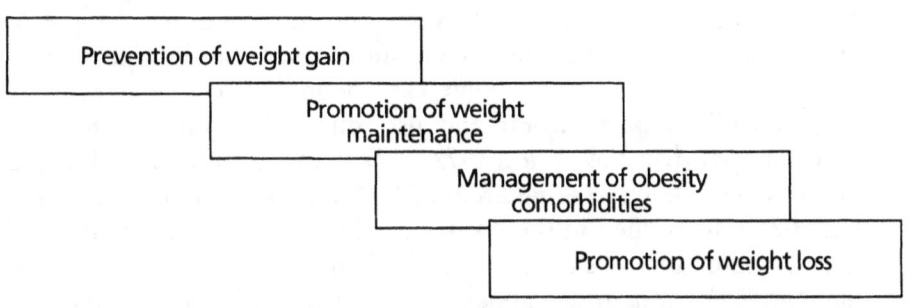

WHO 98269

The diagram shows the broad range of overlapping activities that are an integral part of obesity management. The size of each element indicates its relative contribution to the effective control of obesity.

[a] Adapted from reference *1* with the permission of the publisher Churchill Livingstone.

- The proportion of the population that is either overweight or obese in many developed countries is now so large that there are no longer sufficient health care resources to offer treatment to all (*13*).

- In developing countries, limited resources will quickly be exhausted by the need for expensive and technologically advanced treatment for obesity and other NCDs.

8.3.1 *Effectiveness*

Despite the strong justification for prevention strategies outlined above, there has been little comprehensive research on the effectiveness of such strategies. Indeed, only two studies have so far been specifically concerned with preventing weight gain in adults, and the short-term results achieved are not such as to inspire confidence in the ability to prevent obesity (*14, 15*). Furthermore, the fact that obesity rates are rising rapidly and unchecked in almost all parts of the world casts doubt on whether it is even possible to prevent excessive gains in body weight in the long term.

Indirect evidence that obesity-prevention strategies can play a positive role in combating the escalating problem of obesity is therefore of particular importance, and comes from a variety of sources.

Obesity rates are still low in a number of populations around the world, and many people are able to control their weight successfully over long periods. Furthermore, although there has been a consistent secular increase in obesity rates in most countries, such increases in body weight often vary in magnitude between sexes and social classes. This suggests that there are environmental conditions as well as genetic factors that can protect populations, and individuals within populations, from excessive weight gain. For instance, analysis of the NHANES II data from the USA showed that men and people in higher social classes exhibited much smaller increases in body weight between 1976 and 1980 than women and people in lower social classes (*16*). A similar analysis in Finland also found lower rates of increase in mean BMI over the period 1972–1992 in the most highly educated groups (*17*). In fact, in some areas of Finland, the mean BMI actually fell after 1987 in men in the groups of highest and lowest education, and the rates of increase in mean BMI in women in the high and medium education groups appear to be levelling off. In women of the lowest education group, however, mean BMI continues to rise steeply (see Fig. 8.2). These data suggest that it may be possible to prevent further increases in the average weight of the Finnish population if the success achieved with the better educated groups can be extended to the rest of the population.

It is also of interest that the dramatic increase in obesity rates has followed the pattern of similar epidemics of NCDs such as CHD, which are now abating in countries where preventive strategies have been adopted to deal with these conditions. Comprehensive obesity-prevention programmes have been introduced very recently in Singapore and a few other countries, but insufficient time has elapsed for it to be possible to evaluate their long-term success.

Finally, a number of researchers (*18–21*) have shown that the effective management and support of overweight and obese children can significantly reduce the number who continue to have a weight problem in adulthood. The long-term prevention of weight gain in these studies was achieved during the difficult transition periods of childhood and adolescence when weight gain can be a major problem. Furthermore, in a study in which children were treated together with their parents, the children were successful in reducing and maintaining their weight loss while over time the adults returned to their previous body weight (*21*).

8.3.2 *Aims*

It is important to recognize that the concept of obesity prevention does not simply mean preventing normal-weight individuals from becoming obese, but also encompasses a range of strategies that aim to prevent:

— the development of overweight in normal-weight individuals;
— the progression of overweight to obesity in those who are already overweight;

Figure 8.2
**Mean BMI by educational level in men and women from 1972 to 1992 in the
North Karelia and Kuopio areas of Finland[a]**

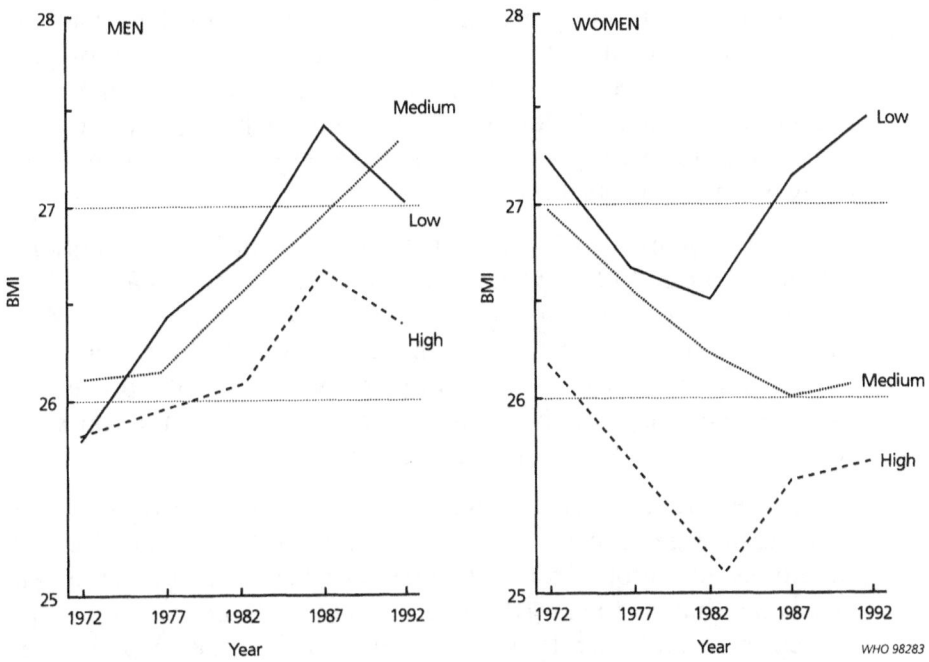

The data show that the mean BMI of Finnish men from low- and high-education groups has
actually declined from a peak in 1987. In Finnish women, the mean BMI declined until 1982
but increased afterwards. Although it appears to be levelling off in women from high- and
medium-education groups, it continues to increase rapidly in low-education groups. These
data suggest that it may be possible to prevent further increases in the average weight of the
Finnish population if the success achieved with the better-educated groups can be extended
to the rest of the population.

[a] Adapted from reference *17* with the permission of the publisher and authors.

— weight regain in those who have been overweight or obese in the
    past but who have since lost weight.

8.3.3 *Levels of preventive action*

The use of the traditional subdivision of prevention into primary,
secondary and tertiary interventions often results in a great deal of
ambiguity and confusion, especially among clinicians. In this scheme,
the objective of primary prevention is to decrease the number of new
cases (incidence), that of secondary prevention is to lower the rate of
established cases in the community (prevalence), and that of tertiary
prevention is to stabilize or reduce the amount of disability associated
with the disorder. It was originally developed for application to acute

conditions with a single identifiable cause but is more difficult to apply to the prevention of a complex, multifactorial condition such as CHD. As a result, attention has usually been focused on individual risk factors, e.g. the primary prevention of CHD has involved national programmes to control blood cholesterol levels, secondary prevention has aimed at reducing further risks in those with existing CHD and elevated blood cholesterol levels, and tertiary prevention has been associated with preventing reinfarction in those who have already had a heart attack.

Similar problems arise when attempting to apply the traditional scheme to obesity prevention. For example, it is not clear whether primary obesity prevention refers to preventing overweight people from becoming obese or whether this is secondary prevention, nor is it clear whether tertiary prevention is concerned with preventing established obesity from becoming more severe or with the control of comorbid conditions such as hypertension.

More recently, an alternative way of classifying preventive interventions has emerged which is more appropriate to chronic multifactorial conditions such as obesity (*1, 22*) and is based on the level of intervention rather than on the target outcome. In the modified version of this concept previously mentioned on p. 155, three levels of prevention (Fig. 8.3) are defined, as follows:

- *Universal/public health prevention* (directed at all members of a community).

- *Selective prevention* (directed at high-risk individuals and groups).

- *Targeted prevention* (directed at those with existing weight problems and those at high risk of diseases associated with overweight).

In this new scheme, only those actions that are carried out before the condition has fully developed are defined as prevention. Many actions aimed at reducing the disability associated with obesity, previously classified as tertiary prevention, are redefined as maintenance interventions.

Universal/public health prevention

Universal/public health prevention programmes are directed at the population or community as a whole, regardless of their current level of risk. The aim is to stabilize the level of obesity in the population, to reduce the incidence of new cases and, eventually, to reduce the prevalence of obesity. However, the most important objective in dealing with a problem of extremes in weight is to reduce the mean weight of the population. The association between the mean level of BMI

Figure 8.3
Levels of prevention measures[a]

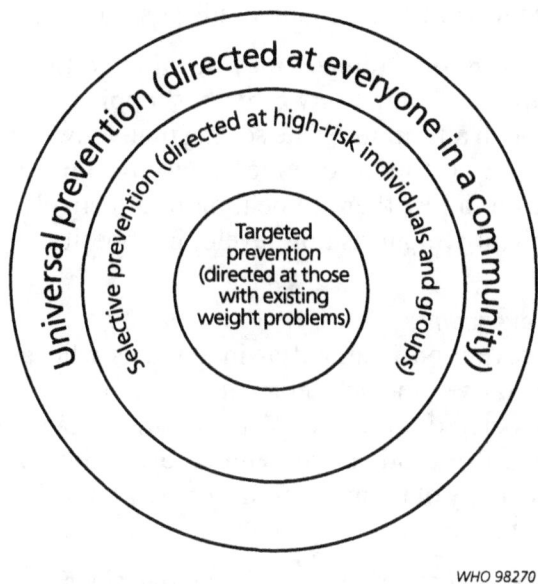

WHO 98270

The diagram shows the three different, but complementary, levels of preventive action for dealing with weight gain and obesity. The very specific targeted-prevention approach is represented by the central circle, the selective preventive approach directed at high-risk individuals and groups is represented by the middle ring, and the broader universal or populationwide prevention approach is represented by the outer ring.

[a] Adapted from reference 1 with the permission of the publisher Churchill Livingstone.

and the prevalence of obesity is discussed in section 9. Other objectives of universal prevention include a reduction in weight-related ill-health, improvements in general diet and PALs, and a reduction in the level of the population risk of obesity.

Such a mass approach to the control and prevention of lifestyle diseases is not always appropriate, and has been criticized for requiring everyone, whether at high or low risk, to make the same changes (23). In the prevention of overweight and obesity, however, where the prevalence of the condition is already extremely high and a large proportion of the population is at high risk, universal approaches have the potential to be the most cost-effective form of prevention (24).

Selective prevention
Selective prevention measures are aimed at subgroups of the population who are at high risk of developing obesity. High-risk subgroups (identified in section 7) are characterized by genetic, biological or

other factors associated with an increased risk of obesity. This risk may be limited in time, as in certain vulnerable life stages, or it may be a lifelong concern, e.g. a genetic predisposition to weight gain.

Selective prevention strategies may be initiated through schools, colleges, workplaces, community centres, shopping outlets and primary care, or through any appropriate setting that allows access to high-risk groups. The aim is to improve the knowledge and skills of groups of people so as to allow them to deal more effectively with the factors that place them at high risk of developing obesity.

Targeted prevention

Targeted prevention is aimed at individuals who are already overweight and those who are not yet obese but in whom biological markers associated with excessive fat stores have been identified. These are high-risk individuals, and failure to intervene at this stage will result in many of them becoming obese and suffering the resulting ill-health in the future.

The primary objectives of the targeted prevention of obesity are limited to the prevention of further weight gain and to the reduction of the number of people who develop obesity-related comorbidities. Patients recruited to targeted prevention programmes will already have some weight-related problems and require intensive individual or small-group preventive intervention. Individuals at high risk of developing obesity comorbidities such as CVD, NIDDM and arthritis are a key target for this prevention strategy. Preventing overweight children from becoming obese adults is a form of targeted prevention.

8.3.4 Integrating obesity prevention into efforts to prevent other noncommunicable diseases

There is much to be gained from incorporating the objectives of obesity prevention into the strategies and programmes for controlling other NCDs. Thus overweight and obesity are important contributors to the risk of several NCDs, the risk increasing with the increase in excess body weight. When obesity and overweight coexist with other NCD risks, the effect is multiplicative (section 4). In addition, dietary modification and PALs are key factors in preventive programmes for both obesity and NCDs, while a number of countries already have NCD prevention programmes that deal with matters relevant to obesity prevention.

WHO has repeatedly emphasized the global importance of obesity and other NCDs during periods of economic transition. Over the past decade, WHO programmes such as the INTERHEALTH project

(Integrated Programme for the Prevention and Control of Noncommunicable Diseases), the CINDI programme (Community Interventions in Noncommunicable DIseases) and the MONICA project for CVD risk-factor monitoring have been important examples of an integrated (horizontal) approach to the NCD epidemic. They are all based on the recognition that all NCDs have a number of common risk factors, necessitating an integrated approach to their prevention, particularly in view of the problem of funding priorities resulting from the emergence of devastating communicable diseases, such as AIDS and Ebola virus disease, and the re-emergence of tuberculosis.

In developed countries, overweight and obesity are seen predominantly in the socioeconomically disadvantaged segments of the population. Public health measures to control NCDs are still inadequate and equity considerations make the introduction of such measures a high priority. The prevention of obesity, in parallel with existing efforts to control other risk factors for NCDs, should provide better control of these diseases. However, such strategies should focus more on obesity *per se* rather than treating it as just another risk factor for NCDs.

In developing countries, where nutritional deficiency disorders and the emerging epidemic of NCDs require attention at the same time, integrated activities designed to meet multiple demands are likely to be of greatest benefit. The prevention of NCDs, including overweight and obesity, should be a public health priority since limited resources will quickly be exhausted by the demand for expensive and technologically advanced curative care, especially in countries in transition. Furthermore, the expected reversal of the social gradient associated with the NCD epidemic will pose insurmountable problems of equity and access to health in these countries.

8.4 Dealing with individuals with existing overweight and obesity

Although prevention potentially offers the most effective long-term approach to the management of obesity, more intensive interventions are also required to deal with the immediate weight and health problems of individuals who are currently obese (see also section 10). As indicated in Chapter 3, such people are alarmingly numerous in most developed and many developing countries. Effective management strategies to deal with them require coordinated and programmed care offered throughout the community and health care services, with the emphasis on weight maintenance, the management of obesity comorbidities and weight loss.

8.4.1 *The current situation*

Given the high prevalence rates of obesity and the well developed national health care systems in many countries, it would seem reasonable to assume that well coordinated and systematic management services exist to deal with obesity. However, the current situation is far removed from this ideal.

In a preliminary survey, Deslypere examined obesity-management approaches in existing national health care services in Australia and in a number of countries in South America, South-East Asia and Europe.[1] A wide variation in obesity care services was found; very few countries had a coherent and comprehensive range of services capable of providing the level of care required to manage obese patients effectively. This is in stark contrast to the situation with regard to other chronic diseases such as NIDDM and CHD, where integrated care is frequently provided through primary health care services.

The Czech Republic, where a five-year plan for the prevention and management of obesity has been established, provides a welcome exception to the rule (V. Hainer, personal communication). A wide range of therapies including diet, exercise, behaviour modification, drug therapy and surgery are currently employed for the treatment of obese patients. Mild-to-moderate obesity is dealt with through weight-reduction clubs, while moderate obesity with comorbidities is treated in obesity outpatient clinics. Severely obese patients are referred to specialist university obesity clinics. Internists receive postregistration training in the care of obese patients, and an obesity-management handbook has been prepared for nurses and another is being prepared for family doctors. Obesity specialists are also involved in the training of counsellors for weight-loss clubs.

8.4.2 *Knowledge and attitudes of health professionals*

Several studies have shown that family doctors and other primary health care professionals have incomplete, confused and occasionally incorrect knowledge of obesity and nutrition (*25–27*). Often the basic facts about weight control are understood, but confusion abounds in relation to how best to manage and advise patients or the public (*28*). Certain genetic and metabolic disorders that lead to the development of obesity are often given undue prominence in discussions in medical textbooks about weight gain and

---

[1] Deslypere JP, ed. *The primary health care–specialist interface*, 1996. Background paper prepared by Primary Health Care–Specialist Interface subgroup of the International Obesity Task Force.

obesity. However, in practice these conditions are very rare and only a tiny proportion of overweight and obesity in patients can be attributed to such causes. This is a major problem, as family doctors are considered by the general public to be the most reliable and credible source of health information (29) and are consulted about weight loss more often than any other health professional (30). Obesity is not a common subject in the prequalification training of health care workers (31–33) and opportunities for postregistration training are usually limited. National obesity societies have generally not taken an active role in the training of health professionals.

Although there has been only a limited assessment in the medical literature of the current attitudes of health professionals, a number of studies in industrialized countries indicate that the current situation is far from satisfactory. The majority of health professionals are pessimistic about their ability to help patients to lose weight by persuading them to change their lifestyles, and many consider obesity management to be frustrating, time-consuming and pointless (34, 35). Although health professionals appear to be well informed about the causes of obesity, many have negative and even derogatory stereotypes of the obese, and especially of the morbidly obese (36–39). Obesity is not generally regarded as a serious medical condition, so that many doctors fail to advise and treat the majority of their obese patients. Obesity tends to be treated only when a comorbidity is present, rather than before it develops or is exacerbated by the obese state (34). Recently, a study was carried out in Germany of the frequency with which the diagnosis "overweight" or "obesity" was entered in outpatient medical records; despite the high prevalence of overweight and obesity in Germany, they were mentioned in the records of only a very small percentage of patients and usually only when accompanied by another chronic condition (40). Even when doctors are aware of the importance of obesity management and monitoring, they often have limited time and resources to devote to such activities (29).

Other health professionals actively involved in the management of obesity include nurses and, in some countries, dietitians. However, although they provide more comprehensive weight management advice than medical doctors (41), the advice does not appear to be any better or more effective than the advice provided by doctors. Confidence in their ability to assist people to lose weight and to maintain weight loss is low among nurses (42), and even dietitians doubt that their current efforts to deal with obesity (43) are effective. Negative attitudes towards obesity and the obese also appear to exist among both nurses (*44*) and dietitians (*39*). Furthermore, in many countries (particularly in eastern Europe) the profession of dietitian is not well established and there are no opportunities for tertiary education in dietetics. Dietary advice is often provided by "dietary assistants" or "diet nurses" who have received no formal training at all. In Sweden, however, nurses can receive further training to become "dietetically competent" and their efficacy in weight management has been demonstrated (*45*).

8.4.3 *Improving the situation*

There is an urgent need to improve the training of all health care workers involved in the management of obese patients. This is important not only to raise the level of knowledge and skills in obesity-management strategies but also to help to overcome the negative attitude that many health professionals have towards obesity and the obese.

It is clear that the rational development of coordinated health care services for the management of overweight and obese patients is needed in all areas of the world. Primary health care services should play the dominant role, but hospital and specialist services are also required for dealing with the more severe cases and the major associated life-threatening complications. Good communications between the different types of health care service are essential.

The concept of "shared care", which involves the formal integration of general medical and specialist services to provide comprehensive services for patients, is finding favour for the management of many other chronic conditions, particularly NIDDM (*46, 47*). Richman et al. evaluated a shared-care obesity management programme involving both general practitioners and a hospital-based specialist obesity service, and found that obese patients managed in such a setting achieved better weight loss in the short term and had lower drop-out rates than similar patients attending a specialist service based at a hospital (*48*).

It is recognized that improvements in obesity-management services will make large demands on resources from all areas of health care, not least because of the widespread nature of the obesity problem. However, if sufficient resources are allocated to the prevention and effective management of weight gain, it should be possible to make significant savings in other areas where obesity is an important underlying cause of morbidity. It has also been shown that an increase in BMI is associated with a concomitant rise in the length of patient hospital stays, medical consultations and demand for medication (*40,*

49, 50). Thus, preventing weight gain and obesity is likely to be more effective in the long term than treating its consequences once it has developed.

8.5 Partnerships for action on obesity

Whether strategies for controlling overweight and obesity are based on the promotion of healthy diets, on increasing levels of physical activity, or on both, they cannot be seen as the sole responsibility of any one sector. To be effective, strategies must be multisectoral and involve the active participation of governments, the food industry/ trade, the media and consumers. Furthermore, they provide an excellent opportunity for the synergistic interaction between government policies on nutrition and NCD control.

8.5.1 *Shared responsibility*

The concept of shared responsibility for the prevention and management of obesity is illustrated in Fig. 8.4, which shows how strategies to promote an appropriate diet and physical activity involve coordinated action by all the sectors concerned.

Promoting healthy diets
The promotion of healthy diets that are low in fat, high in complex carbohydrates and contain large amounts of fresh fruit and vegetables should be a priority in obesity prevention. Although it is consumers who ultimately choose which foods to consume, their choices are influenced by a number of factors such as experience, custom, availability and cost. These factors, in turn, are affected by the actions of government, the food industry and the media. Food availability, for example, depends on the capacity of industry to produce and deliver products to the consumer at affordable prices, and to promote them appropriately, as well as on government policy on food standards, and on subsidies and taxes on food products.

Consumption of a high-fat diet may reflect government policies on the control of food quality, the advertising of high-fat products by the food industry and the media, ready access to processed high-fat fast foods, lifestyles that favour the convenience of preprepared meals, and excessive consumption driven by the pleasant mouth-feel of fat when eaten.

The shared responsibilities of governments, the food industry, the media and consumers, outlined above, offer multiple sites for intervention. Appropriate targets for nutrition strategies identified by FAO and WHO (*51–53*) include consumer education and protection,

Figure 8.4
Healthy weight for all — a shared responsibility[a]

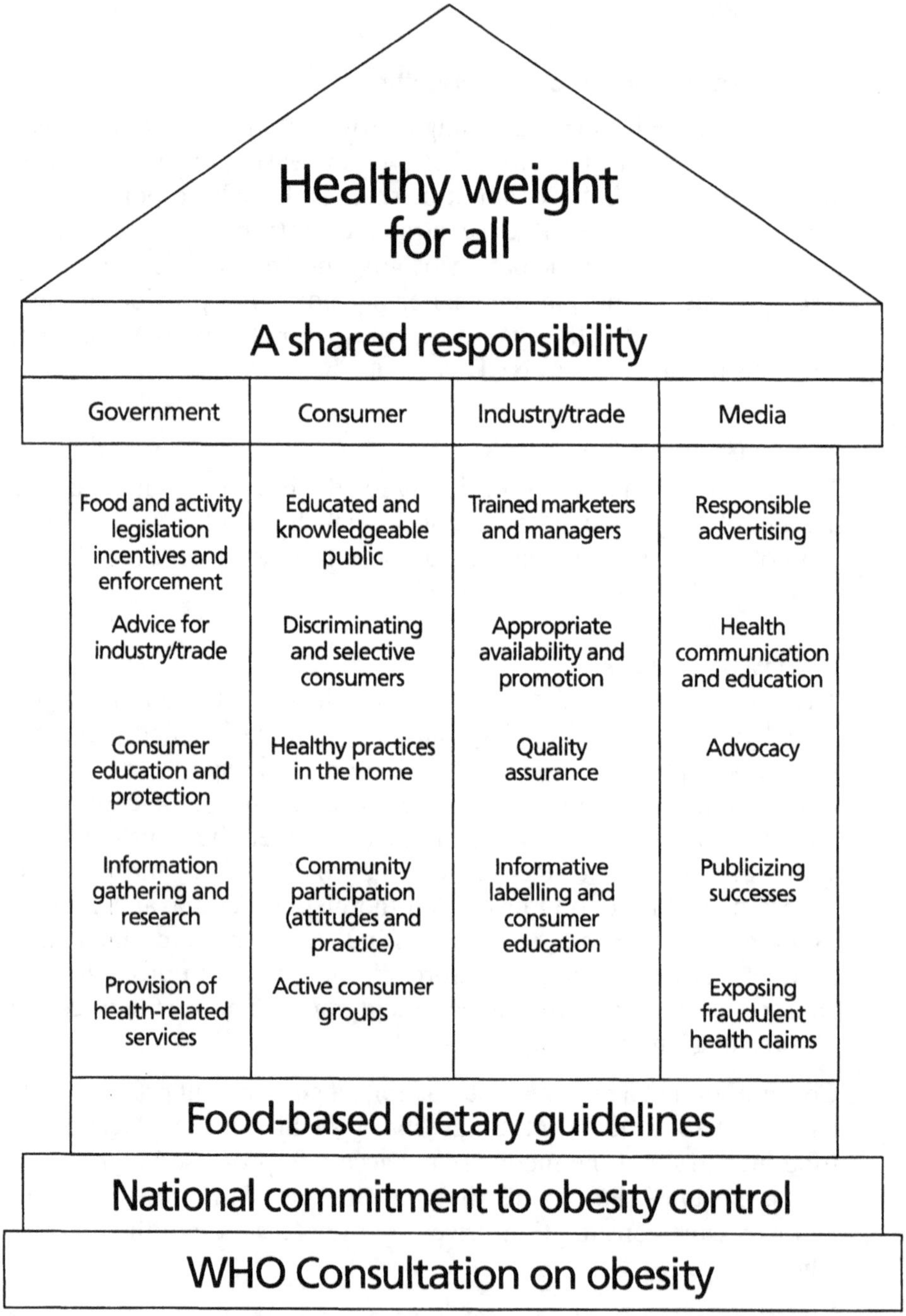

Healthy weight for all

A shared responsibility

Government	Consumer	Industry/trade	Media
Food and activity legislation incentives and enforcement	Educated and knowledgeable public	Trained marketers and managers	Responsible advertising
Advice for industry/trade	Discriminating and selective consumers	Appropriate availability and promotion	Health communication and education
Consumer education and protection	Healthy practices in the home	Quality assurance	Advocacy
Information gathering and research	Community participation (attitudes and practice)	Informative labelling and consumer education	Publicizing successes
Provision of health-related services	Active consumer groups		Exposing fraudulent health claims

Food-based dietary guidelines

National commitment to obesity control

WHO Consultation on obesity

WHO 98271

[a] Adapted from Figure 1 in reference 52

the development and implementation of dietary guidelines, food labelling, nutrition education in schools and efforts to ensure truth in advertising. The food industry plays an important role in the development and promotion of affordable healthy products, while the media are crucial in advocating change, publicizing successes and exposing fraudulent health claims. Governments are responsible for supporting research and collecting information on dietary intake and the nutritional status of the population through epidemiological investigations and surveillance. Programmes aimed at improving the nutritional well-being of people, in particular that of the groups at greatest risk, should be supported through the allocation of adequate resources by both the public and private sectors so as to ensure their sustainability.

Promoting increased physical activity

Greater emphasis on improved opportunities for physical activity is clearly needed, especially in view of the conditions associated with increased urbanization and the parallel increase in time devoted to sedentary pursuits. The provision of convenient and safe exercise facilities, the allocation of time for exercise, a media focus on the role of physical activity in health promotion, workplace interventions aimed at increasing such activity, and consumer education are all methods of increasing energy expenditure.

As with diet quality, PALs depend on the interaction of the influences of many factors that can either promote or restrict activity. However, current environmental conditions in modern societies invariably favour sedentary lifestyles. Opportunities for children to walk/cycle to school or to play outside the home are profoundly affected by factors such as traffic policy and public safety, but schools also need to actively promote physical activity by incorporating a variety of recreational activities into their curricula. Community facilities and town planning policies should facilitate everyday walking and exercise by adults and children, and traffic policies and workplace practices should help to promote sustained physical activity throughout life.

8.5.2 Coordination of government policies

Strategies to improve the prevention and management of overweight and obesity, as well as their comorbidities, provide an opportunity, as previously mentioned, for the synergistic interaction between national policies on nutrition and NCD control. Goals and strategies recommended for obesity control, such as the monitoring of weight status and the promotion of healthy diets and active lifestyles, should be an integral and important part of policies on nutrition and NCD control. The development and effective implementation of such policies require the active participation of the government agencies responsible for education and agriculture.

References

1. Gill TP. Key issues in the prevention of obesity. *British Medical Bulletin*, 1997, **53**:359–388.

2. Kayman S, Bruvold W, Stern JS. Maintenance and relapse after weight loss in women: behavioral aspects. *American Journal of Clinical Nutrition*, 1990, **52**:800–807.

3. Garner DM, Wooley SC. Confronting the behavioural and dietary treatments for obesity. *Clinical Psychological Reviews*, 1991, **11**:573–578.

4. Weintraub M et al. Long-term weight control study. I (weeks 0 to 34). The enhancement of behavior modification, caloric restriction, and exercise by fenfluramine plus phentermine versus placebo. *Clinical Pharmacology and Therapeutics*, 1992, **51**:586–594.

5. Weintraub M et al. Long-term weight control study. II (weeks 34 to 104). An open-label study of continuous fenfluramine plus phentermine versus targeted intermittent medication as adjuncts to behavior modification, caloric restriction, and exercise. *Clinical Pharmacology and Therapeutics*, 1992, **51**:595–601.

6. Weintraub M et al. Long-term weight control study. III (weeks 104 to 156). An open-label study of dose adjustment of fenfluramine and phentermine. *Clinical Pharmacology and Therapeutics*, 1992, **51**:602–607.

7. Weintraub M et al. Long-term weight control study. IV (weeks 156 to 190). The second double-blind phase. *Clinical Pharmacology and Therapeutics*, 1992, **51**:608–614.

8. Weintraub M et al. Long-term weight control study. V (weeks 190 to 210). Follow-up of participants after cessation of medication. *Clinical Pharmacology and Therapeutics*, 1992, **51**:615–618.

9. Weintraub M, Sundaresan PR, Cox C. Long-term weight control study. VI. Individual response patterns. *Clinical Pharmacology and Therapeutics*, 1992, **51**:619–633.

10. Weintraub M, Sundaresan PR, Cox C. Long-term weight control study. VII (weeks 0 to 210). Serum lipid changes. *Clinical Pharmacology and Therapeutics*, 1992, **51**:634–641.

11. Higgins M et al. Benefits and adverse effects of weight loss. Observations from the Framingham Study. *Annals of Internal Medicine*, 1993, **119**:758–763.

12. Pi-Sunyer FX. Medical hazards of obesity. *Annals of Internal Medicine*, 1993, **119**:655–660.

13. James WPT. The epidemiology of obesity. In: Chadwick DJ, Cardew GC, eds. *The origins and consequences of obesity*. Chichester, Wiley, 1996:1–16 (Ciba Foundation Symposium 201).

14. **Forster JL et al.** Preventing weight gain in adults: a pound of prevention. *Health Psychology*, 1988, 7:515–525.

15. **Jeffery RW, French SA.** Preventing weight gain in adults: design, methods and one year results from the Pound of Prevention Study. *International Journal of Obesity and Related Metabolic Disorders*, 1997, 21:457–464.

16. **Kuczmarski RJ.** Prevalence of overweight and weight gain in the United States. *American Journal of Clinical Nutrition*, 1992, 55(Suppl.):495S–502S.

17. **Pietinen P, Vartiainen E, Männisto S.** Trends in body mass index and obesity among adults in Finland from 1972 to 1992. *International Journal of Obesity and Related Metabolic Disorders*, 1996, 20:114–120.

18. **Dietz WH.** Therapeutic strategies in childhood obesity. *Hormone Research*, 1993, 39(Suppl. 3):86–90.

19. **Flodmark CE et al.** Prevention of progression to severe obesity in a group of obese schoolchildren treated with family therapy. *Pediatrics*, 1993, 91:880–884.

20. **Davis K, Christoffel KK.** Obesity in preschool and school-age children: treatment early and often may be best. *Archives of Pediatrics and Adolescent Medicine*, 1994, 148:1257–1261.

21. **Epstein LH et al.** Ten-year outcomes of behavioral family-based treatment for childhood obesity. *Health Psychology*, 1994, 13:373–383.

22. US Institute of Medicine. *Reducing risks for mental disorders: frontiers for preventive intervention research.* Washington, DC, National Academy Press, 1994 (Report of the Committee on Prevention of Medical Disorders Division).

23. **Oliver MF.** Should we not forget about mass control of coronary risk factors? *Lancet*, 1983, ii:37–38.

24. **Stunkard AJ.** Prevention of obesity. In: Brownell KD, Fairburn CG, eds. *Eating disorders and obesity: a comprehensive handbook.* London, Guilford Press, 1995:572–576.

25. **Porteous J.** *Nutrition knowledge, attitudes and practices of New South Wales general practitioners. (Nutrition fellowship report).* Melbourne, Royal Australian College of General Practitioners, 1988.

26. **Francis J et al.** Would primary health care workers give appropriate dietary advice after cholesterol screening? *British Medical Journal*, 1989, 298:1620–1622.

27. **Haines AP, Sanders TAB.** Dietary advice for lowering plasma cholesterol. *British Medical Journal*, 1989, 298:1594–1595.

28. **Murray S et al.** Study of dietetic knowledge among members of the primary health care team. *British Journal of General Practice*, 1993, 43:229–231.

29. **Hiddink GJ et al.** Nutrition guidance by primary-care physicians: perceived barriers and low involvement. *European Journal of Clinical Nutrition*, 1995, 49:842–851.

30. **Crawford D, Worsley A.** Dieting and slimming practices of South Australian women. *Medical Journal of Australia*, 1988, 148:325–328.

31. **Gray J, ed.** *Nutrition in medical education. Report of the British Nutrition Foundation's Task Force on Clinical Nutrition.* London, British Nutrition Foundation, 1983.

32. Royal Society of Medicine Forum on Food and Health. Teaching nutrition to medical students. *Journal of the Royal Society of Medicine*, 1988, **81**:176–178.

33. **Campbell LV, Welborn TA.** Current teaching about obesity in Australian universities. *Medical Journal of Australia*, 1994, **160**:583–584.

34. **Orleans CT et al.** Health promotion in primary care: a survey of US family practitioners. *Preventive Medicine*, 1985, **14**:636–647.

35. **Cade J, O'Connell S.** Management of weight problems and obesity: knowledge, attitudes and current practice of general practitioners. *British Journal of General Practice*, 1991, **41**:147–150.

36. **Blumberg P, Mellis LP.** Medical students' attitudes toward the obese and the morbidly obese. *International Journal of Eating Disorders*, 1985, **4**:169–175.

37. **Price JH et al.** Pediatricians' perceptions and practices regarding childhood obesity. *American Journal of Preventive Medicine*, 1989, **5**:95–103.

38. **Wiese HJ et al.** Obesity stigma reduction in medical students. *International Journal of Obesity and Related Metabolic Disorders*, 1992, **16**:859–868.

39. **Oberrieder H et al.** Attitudes of dietetic students and registered dietitians towards obesity. *Journal of the American Dietetic Association*, 1995, **95**:914–916.

40. **Hauner H, Köster I, von Ferber L.** Frequency of "obesity" in medical records and utilization of out-patient health care by "obese" subjects in Germany. An analysis of health insurance data. *International Journal of Obesity and Related Metabolic Disorders*, 1996, **20**:820–824.

41. **Hopper D, Barker ME.** Dietary advice, nutritional knowledge and attitudes towards nutrition in primary health care. *Journal of Human Nutrition and Dietetics*, 1995, **8**:279–286.

42. **Hoppé R, Ogden J.** Practice nurses' beliefs about obesity and weight related interventions in primary care. *International Journal of Obesity and Related Metabolic Disorders*, 1997, **21**:141–146.

43. **Jones F.** *An investigation of the current practices and opinions of dietitians in the dietary treatment of obesity.* [B.Sc. Honours project.] Edinburgh, Queen Margaret College, 1994.

44. **Brink PJ.** Challenging commonly held beliefs about obesity. *Clinical Nursing Research*, 1992, **1**:418–429.

45. **Bitzen PO et al.** Efficacy of dietary regulation in primary health care patients with hyperglycaemia detected by screening. *Diabetic Medicine*, 1988, **5**:640–647.

46. **Kopelman P, Keable-Elliott D.** An inner city district diabetic care scheme. *Diabetic Medicine*, 1990, **7**:558–560.

47. **Hoskins PL et al.** Sharing the care of diabetic patients between hospital and general practitioners; does it work? *Diabetic Medicine*, 1992, **10**:81–86.

48. **Richman RM et al.** A shared care approach in obesity management: the general practitioner and a hospital based service. *International Journal of Obesity and Related Metabolic Disorders*, 1996, **20**:413–419.

49. **Häkkinen U.** The production of health and the demand for health care in Finland. *Social Science and Medicine*, 1991, **33**:225–237.

50. **Seidell J, Deerenberg I.** Obesity in Europe: prevalence and consequence for use of medical care. *PharmacoEconomics*, 1994, **5**(Suppl. 1):38–44.

51. *Food safety issues: guidelines for strengthening a national food safety programme*. Geneva, World Health Organization, 1996 (unpublished document WHO/FNU/FSU/96.2; available on request from Food Safety, World Health Organization, 1211 Geneva 27, Switzerland).

52. *Promoting appropriate diets and healthy lifestyles: a theme paper prepared for the International Conference on Nutrition*. Rome, Food and Agriculture Organization of the United Nations, 1992 (unpublished document PREPCOM/ICN/92/INF/10, available on request from Department of Nutrition for Health and Development, World Health Organization, 1211 Geneva 27, Switzerland).

53. *Nutrition and development: a global assessment*. Geneva, World Health Organization, 1992 (unpublished document ICN/92/INF/5, available on request from Department of Nutrition for Health and Development, World Health Organization, 1211 Geneva 27, Switzerland).

Prevention and management of overweight and obesity in populations: a public health approach

Introduction

Obesity is a public health problem and must therefore be seen from a population or community perspective. Health problems that affect the well-being of a major proportion of the population are unlikely to be effectively controlled by strategies in which the emphasis is on individuals. Public health action is based on the principle that promoting and protecting the health of the population requires an integrated approach encompassing environmental, educational, economic, technical and legislative measures, together with a health care system oriented towards the early detection and management of disease.

A public health approach to obesity concentrates on the weight status of the population as a whole, in contrast to interventions that deal exclusively with factors influencing the body fatness of individuals. In many developed and developing countries, underprivileged minority groups have to bear a disproportionally heavy burden of higher than average levels of obesity. Thus, in efforts to remove inequalities in health status as one of the main aims of public health, it is necessary to consider the causes that make particular groups more vulnerable to weight gain.

This section deals with the need to develop population-based strategies that tackle the environmental and societal factors identified in section 7 as being implicated in the development of obesity. This is a major area for action in the effective prevention of the global epidemic of obesity. The key issues include the following:

- Obesity is a major global public health problem, and must therefore be approached from a public health standpoint.

- As already mentioned, a public health approach to obesity concentrates on the weight status of the population as a whole in contrast to other interventions that deal exclusively with factors influencing body fatness.

- As the average BMI of a population increases above 23, the prevalence of obesity in that population increases at an even faster rate (see p. 178). A population median BMI range of 21–23 is thought to be the optimum from the point of view of minimizing the level of obesity; adult populations in developing countries are likely to gain greater benefit from a median BMI of 23, whereas those in affluent societies with more sedentary lifestyles are likely to gain greater benefit from a median BMI of 21.

- Appropriate public health strategies to deal with obesity should be aimed both at improving the population's knowledge about obesity and its management and at reducing the exposure of the community to an obesity-promoting environment.

- The two priorities in public health interventions aimed at preventing the development of obesity should be: (1) increasing levels of physical activity; and (2) improving the quality of the diet available within the community. The approaches adopted will depend on the population, and especially its economic circumstances.

- In the past, public health intervention programmes have had limited success in dealing with rising obesity rates, although the results of some countrywide "lifestyle programmes" are encouraging. However, few programmes have concentrated on obesity as a major outcome or have attempted to address environmental influences.

- Current obesity-prevention initiatives need to be evaluated, their limitations recognized, and their designs improved. Lessons learned from public health campaigns on other issues can be used to improve public health campaigns on obesity.

- The prevention and management of obesity are not solely the responsibility of individuals, their families, health professionals or health service organizations; a commitment by all sectors of society is required.

- Public health strategies intended to improve the prevention and management of obesity should aim to produce an environment that supports improved and appropriate eating habits and greater physical activity throughout the entire community. Appropriate action needs to be taken to change urban design, transportation policies, laws and regulations, and school curricula accordingly, provide the necessary economic incentives, introduce catering standards, provide health promotion and education, and promote family food production. Priority should be given to public health action in developing and newly industrialized countries to improve the living conditions of all sectors of society, especially within often neglected aboriginal or native populations.

9.2 Intervening at the population level

The important role of public health action in the control of infectious disease is widely accepted but there is still some scepticism concerning the applicability of this approach to the management of NCDs such as CHD and obesity. The merit of population-level interventions has

Figure 9.1

Relationship between mean BMI and prevalence of obesity in a population[a]

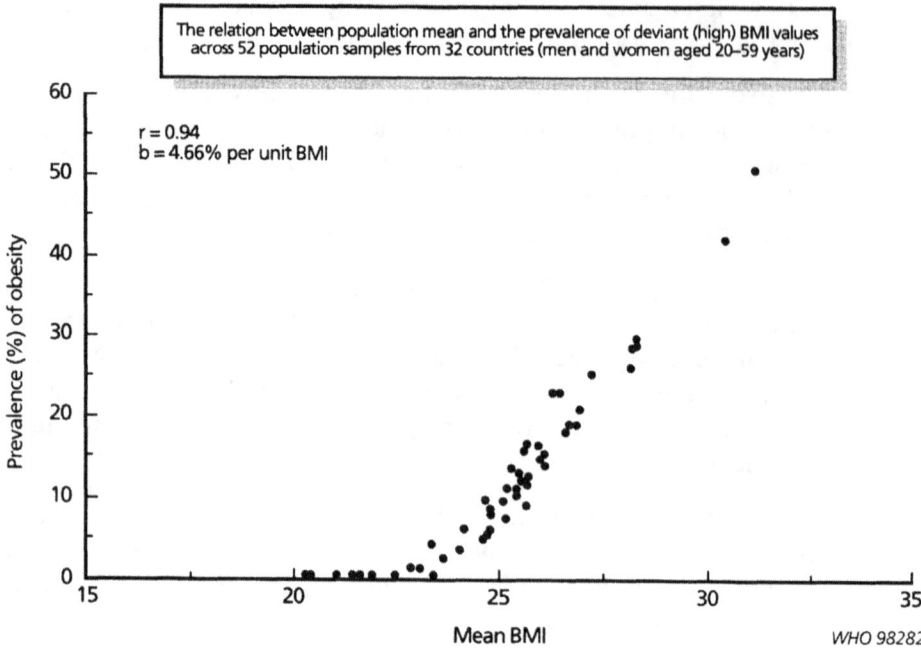

Population mean body weight data from 52 communities in the International Cooperative Study on the Relation of Blood Pressure to Electrolyte Excretion in Populations (INTERSALT) are plotted against the prevalence (%) of obesity; the curve shows the clear relationship between them.

[a] Adapted from reference 3. This figure was first published in: Intersalt: an international study of electrolyte excretion and blood pressure. Results for 24 hour urinary sodium and potassium excretion. *British Medical Journal*, 1988, 297:319–328. Reproduced with the permission of the *British Medical Journal*.

been questioned by some observers because all the members of the community may be urged or obliged to make changes to deal with a problem that currently affects only some of them (*1, 2*). However, if the link between the average and extreme levels of body fatness within a population (Fig. 9.1) is understood, the importance of population-level interventions in obesity can be appreciated, especially as the majority of the adult population in industrialized societies are affected by excess weight gain.

9.2.1 *Relationship between average population BMI and the level of obesity*

The classification of obesity as a BMI ≥30 (section 2) is purely arbitrary. It indicates that health risks are greatly increased above this level of body fatness but not that BMIs below this level are free from such risks. In reality, the population does not consist of two distinct

Figure 9.2
Skewed BMI distribution with increasing population mean BMI[a]

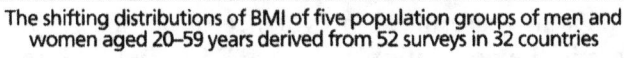
The shifting distributions of BMI of five population groups of men and women aged 20–59 years derived from 52 surveys in 32 countries

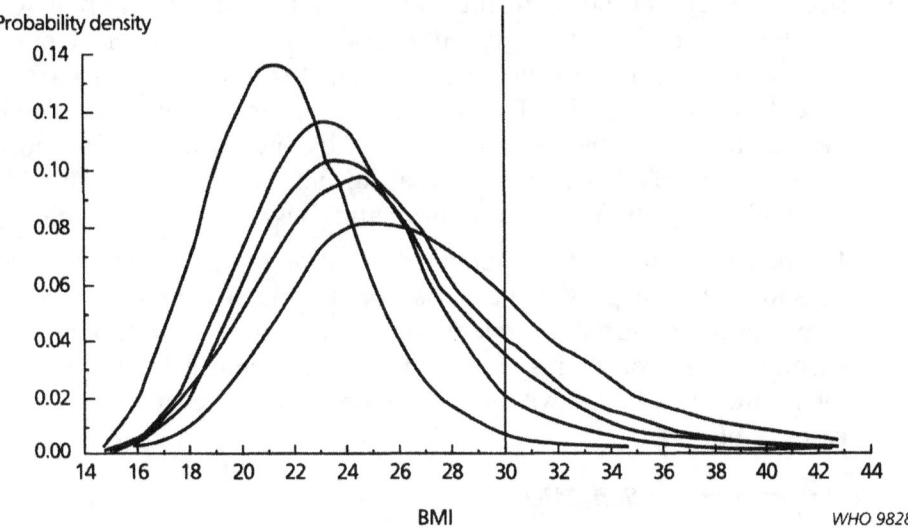

The data from the INTERSALT study show that, as the mean population BMI increases, the level of obesity increases at an even faster rate because of the skewing of the distribution to higher BMIs. Public health interventions seek to prevent this upward shift in mean population BMI.

[a] Adapted from reference 3. This figure was first published in: Intersalt: an international study of electrolyte excretion and blood pressure. Result for 24 hour urinary sodium and potassium excretion. *British Medical Journal*, 1988, 297:319–328. Reproduced with the permission of the *British Medical Journal*.

groups, the obese and the non-obese. The distribution of body fatness within a population ranges from underweight through normal to very obese, and the risks of associated morbidity and mortality begin at relatively low levels of BMI.

The analysis by Rose (3) of the multicountry International Cooperative Study on the Relation of Blood Pressure to Electrolyte Excretion in Populations (INTERSALT) provides a useful evaluation of body weight data from 52 communities. In this study, variations in the distribution of BMI in different adult populations were found that could be predicted from the population mean BMI. When the mean BMI of a population is 23 or below there are few, if any, individuals with a BMI >30. As the BMI distribution of the community shifts to the right (i.e. as mean BMI increases), there is an increased skewing of the data and a flattening of the curve (Fig. 9.2). The result is a greater number of individuals in the population whose BMI exceeds 30.

Perhaps of greatest significance, however, is the accompanying increase in the proportion of adults classified as obese, which takes place at an even faster rate than the increase in average BMI. Rose found a 4.66% increase in the prevalence of obesity for every single unit increase in the population's average BMI above 23, resulting in a strong correlation between the average adult BMI of a population and the proportion of adults with obesity (Fig. 9.1). In the United Kingdom between 1980 and 1993, the mean BMI increased from 24.3 to 25.9 for men and from 23.9 to 25.7 for women. Over this same period, the rates of overweight increased by one-third, whereas those of obesity doubled. This implies that further increases in mean BMI are likely to result in even more dramatic rises in the rates of obesity.

It is believed that, for the effective prevention of obesity, the emphasis should be on preventing a rise in the mean community BMI. Concentrating efforts to prevent and manage obesity on people with existing weight problems (individuals in the right-hand tail of the distribution in Fig. 9.2) will do little to prevent the occurrence of new cases of obesity.

9.2.2 *Optimum population BMIs*

The optimum mean BMI for a population is likely to vary with environmental conditions, e.g. the state of the labour market and the possibility of famine, which differ between developing and developed countries, as well as between urban and rural areas. For example, there are substantial differences in the nutritional status and mean BMI of urban and rural Chinese and Indian communities that reflect vastly different economic and environmental circumstances.

Hazards are associated with both underweight (i.e. BMI <18.5) and overweight (i.e. BMI ≥25). Underweight is a major concern in developing countries and rural areas because work capacity is reduced at BMIs below 18.5 (*4*). Thus, epidemiological studies of national data sets suggest that developing an optimum population BMI will require a trade-off between the two extremes. If the aim is to minimize both the number of adults in a community with a BMI ≥30 (Fig. 9.2) and that of underweight adults with a BMI <18.5, the optimum BMI is about 23. Indeed, the probability of an increasing prevalence of obesity rises markedly above a mean BMI of 23. However, if the aim is to limit the extent of overweight by minimizing the proportion of the population with a BMI ≥25, and there is less concern about limiting the number of adults with a BMI <18.5, a median BMI of 21 is the optimum (*5*).

In industrialized countries there is evidence that a BMI in the lower part of the normal range is associated with the best health outcomes

(6). However, in developing countries, a BMI < 18.5 is not conducive to sustaining prolonged and intensive agricultural work (4).

A median BMI range of 21–23 seems reasonable; adults in developing countries gain greater benefit from a median BMI of 23, and those in affluent societies with more sedentary lifestyles may be better off with a median BMI of 21. National strategies may need to aim at improving the weight status of underweight children and adults in rural communities (target mean BMI 23) and simultaneously at limiting the onset of excessive weight gain in urban communities (whose true optimum target mean BMI may be only 21).

9.2.3 *Will population-based approaches to preventing weight gain lead to increased levels of underweight and eating disorders?*

There has been some concern that strategies aimed at maintaining or reducing the mean BMI of the entire population may result in an increase in the levels of underweight and eating disorders in the community (7, 8). The Rose analysis (3) tends to suggest that those populations with the lowest mean BMI have higher rates of underweight, and that shifting the population distribution of BMI downwards may result in an increase in the numbers of underweight individuals. However, it should be remembered that the data from the INTERSALT study used in Rose's analysis included some from countries where undernutrition remains a significant problem. This is especially relevant for the lowest quintile in Fig. 9.2. Reducing the population mean BMI will not necessarily result in an increase in the proportion of the population classified as underweight or in an increased incidence of eating disorders. Countries that currently exhibit the highest incidence of eating disorders also have the highest population mean BMIs. There is some indication that dieting is associated with an increased risk of eating disorders (9), so that community-level strategies aimed at preventing weight gain in the entire population should be careful to avoid causing the development of eating disorders associated with weight-loss programmes for individuals (10).

9.3 Public health intervention strategies

Two types of public health intervention strategies can generally be used to tackle obesity, namely those that aim to improve the knowledge and skills of individuals in a community, and those that aim to reduce the exposure of populations to the underlying environmental causes of obesity.

9.3.1 *Improving the knowledge and skills of the community*

To date, virtually all public health interventions aimed at the control of obesity in a population have been based on an individual approach.

They have generally relied on the mass media, workplace interventions, school-based programmes and curricula, skills training in a network of clubs and community centres, and community projects to reach a wide audience so as to provide information and promote behaviour change.

While strategies aimed at improving the knowledge and skills of the community have produced impressive results in dealing with many public health problems, this is not true, however, of obesity. This may be because manipulating the diet to prevent public health problems does not induce the same fundamental adaptive responses in eating that are seen when children and adults are underfed in terms of energy. Communities are already generally well aware of the problems associated with obesity, and many individuals are actively attempting to control their weight. Participation rates in this type of obesity control programme are usually high, and many succeed in reducing their weight in the short term. Nevertheless, there is generally little impact on the overall average BMI of the community and a negligible effect on obesity prevalence, so that preventive strategies are obviously of great importance.

9.3.2 *Reducing population exposure to an obesity-promoting environment*

A more effective strategy for dealing with the public health problem of obesity would appear to be one that goes beyond education and deals with those environmental and societal factors that induce the obesity-promoting behaviour of individuals within a population in the first place (see Fig. 7.1). In this way, it may be possible to reduce the exposure of the whole population to social factors that promote obesity, such as the persistent temptation to consume high-fat foods and the convenience of a sedentary lifestyle. Unfortunately, however, such strategies remain relatively unexplored.

9.4 Priority interventions

Regardless of the type of intervention strategy employed to tackle obesity at the population level, two priority interventions important in preventing the development of obesity have been identified in this report, namely increasing levels of physical activity and improving the quality of the diet. The approaches adopted to achieve these aims will depend on the circumstances of the population, and in particular the economic situation. Thus, in developing countries, the main aim of intervention to promote physical activity should be to prevent the reduction in such activity that usually accompanies economic development. In affluent countries, however, the main aim will be to discourage already existing patterns of sedentary behaviour. Likewise, where dietary improvement is concerned, the introduction of new energy-dense foods as a replacement for nutritionally adequate traditional diets should be discouraged in developing countries, whereas the already high consumption of high-fat/energy-dense diets should be reduced in developed ones. Evaluation of interventions is crucial.

9.4.1 *Increasing physical activity*

Interventions aimed at increasing community-wide levels of physical activity (see pp 187–188) are an important means of preventing further increases in the average BMI of a population. Such interventions need to take the following into account:

- Increasing community-wide levels of physical activity has numerous potential benefits for population health in addition to preventing further increases in average BMI, e.g. a reduced risk of NIDDM, CHD and certain cancers.

- Long-term increases in physical activity are more likely to be achieved through environmental changes that increase or maintain incidental daily activity and low-intensity leisure pursuits rather than by encouraging occasional vigorous exercise. The emphasis should be on promoting relatively low-intensity, long-duration physical activity that can be conveniently incorporated into daily life (see also Box 7.2 and pp 117–118). Popular examples of physical activity of this type include walking a dog, gardening, dancing, cycling, home improvement and swimming. Walking in pedestrian precincts rather than depending on car travel and ensuring that some work is done when standing rather than sitting will help to increase daily activity.

- Exercise should also be encouraged, but it should not be presented as requiring excessive physical effort involving boring routines and/ or requiring expensive equipment.

- Activity should be enjoyable in order to encourage regular participation and to discourage sedentary behaviour.

- There is some evidence that physically active children remain active in adult life, so that encouraging young children to take part in a variety of general activities may be especially important.

9.4.2 *Improving the quality of the diet*

Interventions aimed at improving the quality of the diet need to take into account the following important issues relating to dietary energy density and nutrient/energy ratios:

- A major concern associated with the feeding of infants and young children is ensuring that they consume adequate energy. The energy density of traditional diets is often increased by the addition of vegetable oil (taking care not to distort the protein/energy ratio), and children under the age of 2 years should be excluded from any interventions designed to reduce national fat intakes in industrialized countries.

- It is also important to ensure that the nutrient/energy ratio of the diet is adequate, especially in children who may be at risk of micronutrient deficiency. Low nutrient/energy ratios can become a particular problem when the energy content of diets is increased by the addition of fat and refined carbohydrate.

- It is unusual for energy deficiency to arise in adults simply because the bulkiness of their food is such that they are unable to eat enough of it. A more serious problem is the overconsumption of energy-dense diets rich in fat and highly refined products and low in fibre that promote overconsumption and weight gain, especially when eaten by relatively inactive individuals.

Care is therefore needed when both the energy density and the nutrient/energy ratio of diets are examined. The age group targeted in health promotion strategies as well as the normal dietary constituents available to them should be taken into account. When diets are based essentially on unrefined indigenous local foods, and contain a suitable proportion of cereals, pulses, vegetables and affordable animal proteins, there is less likelihood that either their energy density or their nutrient/energy ratios will be inappropriate. Identifying the optimum ranges of both nutrient/energy ratios and energy densities for young children and the corresponding ratios and densities for older children and adults is still difficult.

For information on the national nutrition programmes of Finland and Norway, see pp 188–189.

9.4.3 *Measures for use in evaluating obesity-prevention programmes*

The aim of obesity prevention is to stop the increase in obesity or reduce the number of new cases of this disease in a population. This can be achieved only if rises in the average BMI of the population are prevented.

From a purely scientific viewpoint, the most accurate measures for use in evaluating obesity-prevention programmes are changes in the mean population BMI or in obesity incidence. However, in practical terms, incidence is rarely assessed, and public health authorities are unlikely to accept very small percentage shifts in mean BMI as a significant indicator of public health improvement.

At present, prevalence rates of obesity and its comorbidities are the most commonly used measures of the success or failure of interventions aimed at controlling obesity. However, these have a number of serious limitations when used in isolation. First, the prevalence of obesity within a population is unlikely to decline in the short term; losing weight is not easy and it is unrealistic to expect a large number of obese people to lose sufficient weight to cease to be classified as obese. Second, a long time often elapses before appropriate environmental, societal and behavioural changes are reflected in the population's weight status. Third, estimates of the prevalence of, and trends in, obesity are often unreliable because small sample sizes reduce their accuracy. Finally, the multifactorial etiology of obesity comorbidities limits the use of their prevalence rates as outcome measures for evaluating obesity-prevention programmes because changes in the prevalence of these conditions can occur independently of the population's weight status, e.g. reductions in CHD rates have been achieved as a result of reductions in hypertension and smoking.

A more practical and useful outcome indicator for evaluating obesity prevention would be to combine the assessment of changes in the prevalence of overweight (BMI ≥25) with short-term indicators such as standardized measures of dietary change and of PALs. In fact, prevalence estimates of overweight reflect weight distribution in the population better than estimates of obesity prevalence and are easier to estimate accurately, especially in developing countries with very low rates of obesity. They also account for a significant proportion of the health risks associated with excess weight and body fat. The assessment of mean population BMI and changes in obesity prevalence is also desirable.

9.5 Results of public health programmes for the control of obesity

To date, there have not been any well evaluated and properly organized public health programmes aimed at the population-level management or prevention of obesity. A number of countries have recently developed lifestyle strategies in which the emphasis is on weight control but, except in Singapore, these have not taken the form of controlled trials and so are unlikely to provide any definitive evidence of their impact. The best examples of such trials are community-wide CHD prevention programmes that have included a reduction in BMI as one of the measurable outcomes.

Alternatively, some programmes have targeted those factors identified as important in the development of obesity, namely physical activity and the quality of the diet. However, it is debatable how much can be deduced from the results of such programmes as far as the potential of public health strategies to manage weight is concerned.

9.5.1 *Countrywide public health programmes*

At present, very few countries have a comprehensive populationwide national policy or strategy to deal specifically with the problem of overweight and obesity, in spite of the reports produced in a number of countries, such as Australia (*11*), Canada (*12*) and the United Kingdom (*13*), which have all indicated that this is precisely what is required to tackle obesity effectively. Singapore is one country that has been able to achieve a degree of success in tackling obesity through a system of coordinated healthy lifestyle programmes aimed at specific target groups in the population. The Government of Singapore has an overall strategy that is translated into programmes covering all the stages of life, and including preschool children, schoolchildren, young people and adults. Such programmes rely heavily on community input in their establishment and management (*14*). Recent results of the Trim and Fit programmes (see below) are promising, obesity rates dropping among primary, secondary and junior college students (*15*).

The Trim and Fit programme was launched in 1992 and is aimed at all schoolchildren in Singapore. It combines progressive nutrition changes in school catering, and nutrition education together with regular physical activity in schools. The programme is supported by specialized training for school principals, teachers and canteen workers, as well as by the provision of equipment for improved catering and physical activity. A national monitoring programme to assess fitness and weight status also forms part of this initiative (*16*). Recent results indicate that the number of children successfully completing the fitness tests is increasing annually, and that obesity rates fell from 14.3% in 1992 to 10.9% in 1995 for primary students, from 14.1% to 10.9% for secondary students, and from 10.8% to 6.1% for junior college students (*15*). However, it should be noted that this decline in obesity rates may have been somewhat exaggerated because of the new weight-for-height norms introduced by the Ministry of Health in 1993.

9.5.2 *Communitywide CHD prevention programmes*

Over the last 20 years a handful of well funded, large-scale, communitywide intervention programmes intended to prevent CHD have been conducted, aimed at reducing the level of a number of risk factors, including smoking, high blood pressure, high blood cholesterol and obesity. In-depth evaluation of these programmes and their results has consistently shown that obesity is harder to control than any other risk factor, as indicated for the following five programmes:

- *The Stanford Three Community Project (17) and the Stanford Five City Study (18).* In both of these studies, the mass media and communitywide health education were used to increase awareness and knowledge of CHD and to teach the skills required for appropriate behaviour change to reduce CHD risk (*19*). In both projects, weight reduction and increased physical activity were viewed as methods of facilitating risk factor reduction rather than as outcomes in their own right. The original Three Community Project was successful in preventing weight gain in the treatment groups. In the Five City Study, weight gain in the intervention communities was significantly less than in the control communities (0.57 kg compared with 1.25 kg) over the 6 years. However, the results of repeated surveys of the intervention and control cohort groups showed no differences in the rate of weight gain. Nevertheless, both studies showed significant improvements in blood pressure, cholesterol and smoking rates.

- *The Minnesota Heart Health Program.* This was a relatively unsuccessful CHD intervention programme conducted over 7 years in six matched communities (rural, urban and suburban). The strategies used were similar to those employed in the Stanford studies but the Program was unable to reproduce the improvements in CHD risk factors. However, this intervention was conducted at a time when there were marked secular downward trends in CHD risks in these communities. The 7-year intervention had little impact on obesity. Indeed, BMI showed a strong secular increase despite such innovative weight-control programmes as adult education classes, a workplace weight-control programme, weight loss by correspondence course and a weight-gain-prevention programme (*20*).

- *The North Karelia Project.* Initiated in 1972 in North Karelia, a province in eastern Finland (*21*), this intervention was delivered through the usual mass-media educational, workplace and school-based programmes but included wider community participation in the development and implementation of projects. It set out to integrate the programme into existing, or newly created, services and community infrastructure. In addition, various public health, environmental and structural and legislative measures made healthy behaviours easier to adopt. Despite remarkable reductions in CHD risk factors, which were still declining in 1992 (22), the average BMI and the level of obesity remained similar throughout the project, and similar trends have been observed since its conclusion (23).

- *Mauritius.* In 1987, an NCD intervention project was started by the Government of the developing island country of Mauritius after a population survey revealed high levels of NIDDM and hypertension, and moderately high levels of CHD. An intensive communitywide prevention programme was initiated that made extensive use of the mass media, community, school and workplace health education activities, as well as fiscal and legislative measures designed to encourage a healthy diet, increased exercise, smoking cessation and reduced alcohol intake. After 5 years there had been significant decreases in the prevalence of hypertension, cigarette smoking and heavy alcohol consumption, an appreciable reduction in mean population cholesterol levels, and an improvement in moderate leisure physical activity. However, the levels of overweight (BMI 25–30) and obesity (BMI ≥30) increased by 33% and 56%, respectively, in men and by 19% and 46%, respectively, in women (24).

The following possible reasons for communitywide CHD intervention programmes being disappointing in terms of obesity and weight control have been suggested by Jeffery (20):

- The main emphasis of the programmes was on CHD risk and not obesity. Weight reduction was generally viewed as a method of facilitating risk factor reduction rather than as an outcome in its own right.

- Rapidly rising secular trends in weight may have overwhelmed any effects of interventions aimed at curbing the rise.

- Powerful societal and environmental obesity-promoting factors have developed rapidly in many societies over the last few decades, and the intervention programmes may not have been strong enough or sufficiently well coordinated to overcome them.

- The interventions may not have reached a sufficiently large proportion of the community to have an impact on the weight status of the population as a whole. In many communities, a large percentage are already concerned about weight and are trying to control it, so that even intensive interventions may not increase the number of people actively participating in weight-control programmes.

- The interventions may have been aimed at making too many changes at once (e.g. reducing cholesterol levels, controlling blood pressure, increasing physical activity, stopping smoking, etc.). Health promotion research has shown that campaigns with a more limited objective are often more effective in encouraging behaviour change than those that seek to bring about simultaneous change in several behaviours (*25, 26*).

9.5.3 *Programmes targeting factors important in the development of obesity*

Countrywide programmes aimed at increasing physical activity

Physical inactivity and sedentary behaviour have been identified as two important contributory factors in the development of overweight and obesity (section 7). Increasing communitywide levels of physical activity would therefore appear to be important in preventing further increases in the average BMI of the whole population, in addition to having numerous other potential beneficial effects on its health.

A review by King (*27*) was able to identify only a few well evaluated and truly comprehensive communitywide programmes aimed at increasing levels of physical activity. Such programmes have usually involved a series of interventions targeted at different segments of the population (e.g. health care providers, the elderly, adults in general), have used a variety of channels (print and broadcast media, face-to-face instruction), and have been based in a number of different settings (neighbourhoods, workplaces, schools). However, the degree of integration of these different interventions in reaching the whole population has varied greatly between programmes. Evaluating the success of any such interventions has been hampered by problems associated with the objective assessment of physical activity, by the failure to define the components of physical activity clearly, and by the lack of precise goals in terms of the expected increase in activity.

Evidence from a number of communitywide CHD prevention programmes suggests that intensive intervention can increase participation in physical activity, at least in the short term. This conclusion is supported by the results of a recent nationwide campaign to increase physical activity in Australia. The campaign, called "Exercise — make it a part of your day" was able to demonstrate a significant increase in the level of walking among a sample of the community and increased readiness to undertake further exercise (*28*). These improvements occurred across all social classes and were most marked in the elderly. However, a second campaign, "Exercise — take another step", introduced 1 year later in an attempt to build on the success of the first, was not able to demonstrate any further improvements in levels of activity or willingness to participate (*29*).

Although the improvements achieved by communitywide programmes for increasing physical activity tended to be only short-lived, they
do suggest that participation in physical activity can be increased by
such programmes. Some of the limitations of communitywide CHD
prevention programmes discussed earlier are equally applicable to
programmes intended to increase physical activity. With very few
exceptions, most of the intervention strategies were aimed at improving the awareness of, and motivation to, exercise without tackling the
environmental obstacles to increased participation. The Minnesota
Heart Program did attempt to improve exercise facilities in the community and to involve community groups in establishing their own
committees to review other methods of increasing activity, but most
other programmes relied on interventions based on personal education and behaviour change. In all the programmes, the interventions
were aimed at improving the levels of leisure-time exercise, and did
not attempt to influence factors such as transportation and urban
design that have an impact on occupational and leisure-time daily
activity patterns.

The feasibility of long-term maintenance of increased physical activity and its benefits for obesity prevention remain to be demonstrated
(27, 29).

National nutrition programmes

The energy density and fat content of the food supply have been
identified as the major dietary factors implicated in the development of
obesity (section 7). In many countries, national nutrition programmes
have succeeded in dramatically altering the fatty-acid composition of
diets, and some have also been successful in achieving a small reduction in the intake of total fats. However, very few countries have been
able to reduce total fat intake to the level that would appear to be
necessary to influence the average BMI of the whole population. This
is not surprising, as very few countries have a comprehensive and
integrated national nutrition policy that can direct the actions at all
levels necessary to achieve such a dramatic dietary change.

Two countries that have instituted far-reaching national nutrition
programmes are Finland and Norway. These countries have been able
to reduce national fat intake from 42% to around 34% of total dietary
energy over the last 20 years. It is therefore encouraging to see that
the increase in obesity prevalence is slowing in Finland and that the
mean BMI is stabilizing or even falling in some areas despite simultaneous decreases in levels of physical activity (23) (Fig. 9.3). In Norway, data for all 40–42-year-old men and women recruited to a
countrywide CHD prevention programme (except Oslo) were

Figure 9.3
Changes in mean BMI in men and women in four areas of Finland between 1972 and 1992[a]

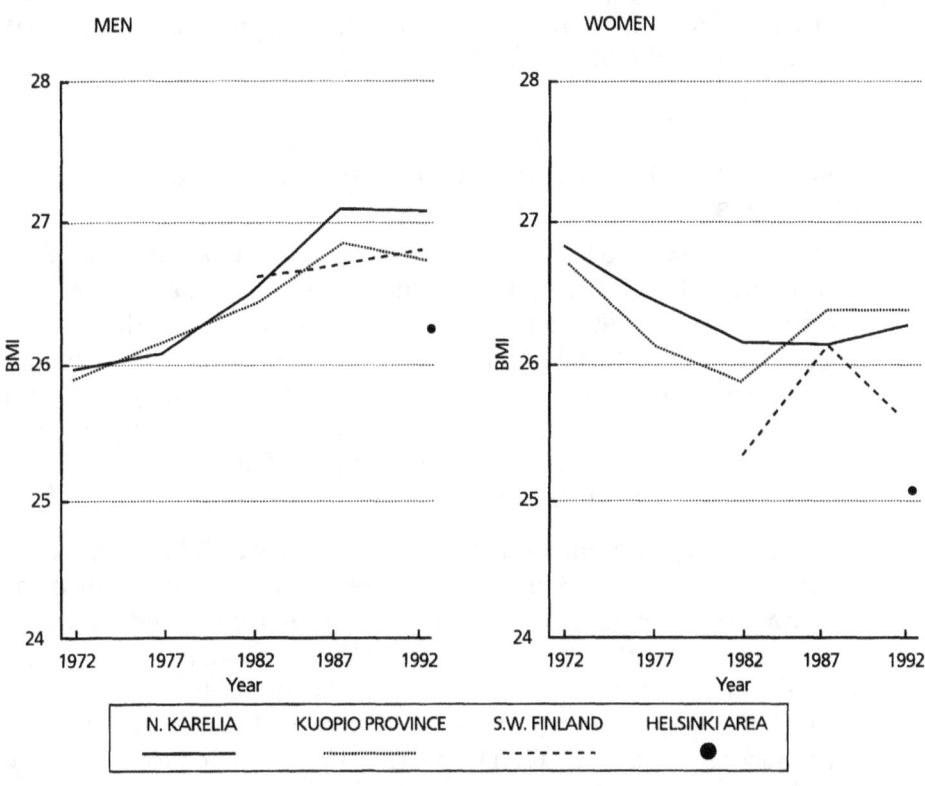

WHO 98280

The curves show that mean BMI for men in North Karelia and Kuopio has stabilized or even fallen since 1987 after rapid rises in the preceding 15 years. The rise in mean BMI for women in the same provinces observed after 1982 also appears to be levelling out. This suggests that the communitywide changes in diet that have occurred in these provinces over the past 25 years may be contributing to a stabilization of population mean BMI.

[a] Adapted from reference 23 with the permission of the publisher and authors.

analysed in a recent study and it was found that obesity rates had decreased slightly in women since the 1960s (30). In Norwegian men, obesity rates remain lower than in other European countries but, in contrast to the Norwegian women, have increased substantially since the 1960s.

9.5.4 *Implications for future public health programmes to control obesity*

What has been demonstrated by these and other lifestyle intervention programmes is that approaches firmly based on the principle of personal education and behaviour change are unlikely to succeed in an environment in which there are plentiful inducements to engage in behaviours that lead to a chronic positive energy imbalance (31).

It would therefore seem appropriate to devote resources to programmes designed to reduce the exposure of the population to obesity-promoting agents by concentrating on environmental factors such as transportation, urban design, advertising and food pricing that promote the availability of high-fat, energy-dense diets and physical inactivity.

9.6 Lessons to be learned from successful public health campaigns

Campaigns that have been relatively successful in dealing with public health problems in the past include those on smoking, wearing seatbelts, drink-driving and immunization. Analyses of these campaigns have helped to identify features that may provide valuable guidance for public health interventions to control obesity. For example, it appears that programmes that involve government, the food industry, the media and the community, and that are of long duration, lead to positive and sustainable change.

Public health programmes on obesity are unlikely to achieve the same spectacular rates of success as those associated with the control of infectious disease; unlike pathogens, it is not feasible to eliminate all the causes of obesity, nor is it a simple matter to isolate and manage the exposure to major disease-promoting factors in the way that the control of smoking and hypertension have contributed to the successful reduction in rates of CHD. Obesity, the consequence of energy imbalance, is more tightly controlled physiologically than other risk factors.

The main features of successful public health campaigns aimed at behaviour change that should be considered in developing public health interventions to control obesity are outlined in Table 9.1 (*32*).

9.7 Public health strategies to improve the prevention and management of obesity

As highlighted in section 7, many features of the modern environment are conducive to a positive energy balance. Traditional foodstuffs are being replaced by high-fat, energy-dense food that is appetizing, packaged attractively, preprocessed for convenience, widely advertised and relatively inexpensive. There is good evidence to suggest that exposure to television food advertising influences food selection among children and adolescents (*37–39*), and in particularly susceptible subgroups (*40*), and convenience foods now account for a substantial proportion of food expenditure in most developed countries. Consumption of convenience foods is also increasing rapidly in devel-

Table 9.1
Main features of successful public health campaigns

Feature of campaign	Example
Adequate duration and persistency	In Finland, even if changes were not spectacular in the first 10 years of the campaign (*22*), recent years have seen marked improvements in CHD risk factors.
A slow and staged approach	Campaigns to change single behaviours, e.g. cigarette smoking, have required a series of strategies over time in order to support the transition from awareness, through motivation to change; experimenting and adopting a change; and maintaining that changed behaviour. This suggests that it is unrealistic to expect rapid changes in complex behaviours such as eating and exercise (*33*).
Legislative action	In some instances, e.g. seat-belt use and drink-driving, legislative action has been necessary to support education campaigns aimed at changing behaviour and attitudes (*34*).
Education	Improved immunization rates for many childhood diseases have required a systematic coordinated approach including both education and regulation. Education can encourage and support a change in behaviour while avoiding the feeling that change is being imposed without reason (*35*).
Advocacy	Strong advocacy from respected elements within all sectors of society has been a key feature of the decrease in smoking rates and in passive smoking (*21*).
Shared responsibility by consumers, communities, food industry and governments	In Portugal, concern for the high prevalences of hypertension and stomach cancer led to a national campaign to reduce the salt content of the diet. This involved an education campaign to reduce salt use in cooking, consumption of salted codfish and salted sausage and, with local bakers, the salt content of bread. Strong local support was obtained from village leaders, doctors and nurses. After 1 year, salt consumption had fallen markedly (by 50%) with a 5-mmHg (0.667-kPa) reduction in average blood pressure (*36*).

oping countries. The Massachusetts Medical Society Committee on Nutrition suggested that fast-food dining has become so well accepted that recommendations that it should be reduced or eliminated are likely to have little or no success (*41*). An effective approach would therefore be to improve both the nutritional quality of the convenience foods available and the eating habits of consumers.

Although recent surveys indicate that involvement in leisure-time physical activity may be increasing, the intensity and duration of such activity is decreasing (42) and participation is often limited by the availability and cost of using facilities. Instead, television viewing has become the major leisure pursuit of children and adults. Furthermore, while road networks expand, there has been little investment in cycle paths or public parks and playing fields. Buildings are designed on the assumption that lifts are preferable to stairs, and there is a common perception that it is unsafe to walk or play in the streets because of the risk of traffic accidents or crime (43). The level of occupational activity has also been declining in recent years because an increasing proportion of the labour force is employed in more sedentary occupations.

9.7.1 *Developed countries*

Since developed countries are characterized by the easy availability of high-fat, energy-dense diets and physical inactivity, it is not surprising that interventions based on education for behaviour change have had limited success in controlling obesity. There is a desperate need for interventions aimed at producing an environment that supports improved eating and physical activity habits throughout the community. This will require a comprehensive and integrated range of strategies in line with the examples shown in Table 9.2. The adoption of such an approach will require general acceptance of the principle that the prevention and management of obesity are not only the responsibility of individuals, their families or health professionals but also require a commitment from all sectors of society. Until this is achieved, strategies for the prevention and management of obesity will remain ineffective.

9.7.2 *Developing and newly industrialized countries*

A number of the possible environmental strategies for obesity control suggested in Table 9.2 are highly sophisticated and assume a certain level of infrastructure that may not exist in developing countries. However, the underlying targets, namely to improve dietary quality and ensure appropriate levels of physical activity, are obviously still relevant and should be incorporated into strategies to prevent the situation from worsening.

As in developed countries, obesity in the developing and newly industrialized countries will not be prevented simply by telling individuals and communities to change their diet and exercise behaviours. What is needed is a radical improvement in the social, cultural and economic environment through the combined efforts of government, the

Table 9.2
Possible environmental strategies for obesity control[a]

Area for action	Example of possible strategies
Urban design and transportation policies	Create pedestrian zones in city centres Construct safe walkways and cycle paths Introduce incentive schemes to encourage use of car parks on the outskirts of cities in conjunction with city public transport (e.g. park and ride) Provide affordable facilities for securing bicycles in cities and public areas Improve public transport (e.g. frequency and reliability of services) Increase safety by improving street lighting Install traffic-calming measures to increase safety of children walking and playing in streets Allocate resources to build and manage community recreation centres Modify building design to encourage use of stairs
Laws and regulations	Improve labelling of food products Limit and regulate advertising to children
Economic incentives	Introduce subsidies for producers of low-energy-dense foods (especially fruits and vegetables) Reduce car tax for those who take public transport to work during the week Provide tax breaks for companies that provide exercise and changing facilities for employees
School curricula	Provide adequate sport and activity areas and facilities, including changing and showering areas Ensure allocation of sufficient curriculum time to physical activity Ensure training in practical food skills for all children
Food and catering	Develop nutrition standards and guidelines for institutional food services and catering (e.g. school meals and workplace catering)
Promotion and education	Promote from an early age a knowledge of food and nutrition, food preparation, and healthy diets and lifestyles through curricula for schoolchildren, teachers, health professionals, and agricultural extension personnel Limit television viewing by children Use the media to promote positive behaviour change (e.g. through television series) Educate the public, especially in areas where food is purchased, on appropriate behaviour change to reduce risk of weight gain Educate the public on the need for collective action to change the environment into one that promotes rather than inhibits exercise and healthy dietary habits Educate the public about important factors in the development of obesity so that victimization of the obese is reduced

Table 9.2
(*Continued*)

Area for action	Example of possible strategies
Family food production	Encourage use of land in towns and cities for "family" growing of vegetables, legumes and other nutrient-rich crops

[a] Adapted from reference *32* with the permission of the publisher Churchill Livingstone.

food industry, the media, communities and individuals. Wider issues, such as the development of national dietary guidelines and the importation, pricing and availability of food, also call for public health action. Improving the standard of living of all sectors of society, and especially of often neglected native or minority populations, should be a priority. The support of international agencies and bodies, such as FAO, UNDP, UNICEF, WHO and the World Bank, as well as nongovernmental organizations is essential.

References

1. Oliver MF. Should we not forget about mass control of coronary risk factors? *Lancet*, 1983, ii:37–38.

2. Atrens DM. The questionable wisdom of a low-fat diet and cholesterol reduction. *Social Science and Medicine*, 1994, **39**:433–447.

3. Rose G. Population distributions of risk and disease. *Nutrition, Metabolism and Cardiovascular Diseases*, 1991, 1:37–40.

4. Shetty PS, James WPT. Functional consequences of low BMI in adults. In: *Body mass index. A measure of chronic energy deficiency in adults*. Rome, Food and Agriculture Organization of the United Nations, 1994 (FAO Food and Nutrition Paper Series, No. 56).

5. James WP, François PJ. The choice of cut-off point for distinguishing normal body weights from underweight or "chronic energy deficiency" in adults. *European Journal of Clinical Nutrition*, 1994, **48**(Suppl. 3):S179–S184.

6. Manson JE et al. Body weight and mortality among women. *New England Journal of Medicine*, 1995, **333**:677–685.

7. Jeffery RW. Population perspectives on the prevention and treatment of obesity in minority populations. *American Journal of Clinical Nutrition*, 1991, **53**(6 Suppl.):S1621–S1624.

8. Allison DB, Engel CN. Obesity prevention: Theoretical and methodological issues. In: Angel A et al., eds. *Progress in obesity research 7*. London, John Libbey, 1996:607–612.

9. Polivy J, Herman CP. Dieting and binging. A causal analysis. *American Psychologist*, 1985, 40:193–201.

10. **Garner DM, Wooley SC.** Confronting the failure of behavioural and dietary treatments for obesity. *Clinical Psychology Review*, 1991, **11**:573–578.

11. *Healthy weight Australia — a national strategy.* Sydney, Australian Society for the Study of Obesity, 1995.

12. Health and Welfare Canada. *Promoting healthy weights: a discussion paper.* Ottawa, Ministry of Supply and Services, Canada, 1988.

13. *Obesity: reversing the increasing problem of obesity in England (a report from the Nutrition and Physical Activity Task Forces).* London, Department of Health, 1995.

14. **Rajan U.** Management of childhood obesity — Singapore perspective. In: Ismael MN, ed. *Proceedings of the first scientific meeting on obesity.* Kuala Lumpur, Malaysian Society for the Study of Obesity (MASSO), 1996, **1**:131–137.

15. *Update on trim and fit programme.* Singapore, Ministry of Education, 1996.

16. *The national healthy lifestyle programme.* Singapore, Ministry of Education, 1994.

17. **Fortmann SP et al.** Effect of health education on dietary behavior: the Stanford Three Community Study: *American Journal of Clinical Nutrition*, 1981, **34**:2030–2038.

18. **Farquhar JW et al.** Effects of communitywide education on cardiovascular disease risk factors: the Stanford Five-City Project. *Journal of the American Medical Association*, 1990, **264**:359–365.

19. **Taylor CB et al.** Effect of long-term community health education on body mass index. *American Journal of Epidemiology*, 1991, **134**:235–249.

20. **Jeffery RW.** Community programs for obesity prevention: the Minnesota Heart Health Program. *Obesity Research*, 1995, 3(Suppl. 2):283S–288S.

21. **Puska P et al.** The community-based strategy to prevent coronary heart disease: conclusions from the ten years of the North Karelia project. *Annual Review of Public Health*, 1985, **6**:147–193.

22. **Vartiainen E et al.** Twenty-year trends in coronary risk factors in north Karelia and in other areas of Finland. *International Journal of Epidemiology*, 1994, **23**:495–504.

23. **Pietinen P, Vartiainen E, Männisto S.** Trends in body mass index and obesity among adults in Finland from 1972 to 1992. *International Journal of Obesity and Related Metabolic Disorders*, 1996, **20**:114–120.

24. **Dowse GK et al.** Changes in population cholesterol concentrations and other cardiovascular risk factor levels after five years of the non-communicable disease intervention programme in Mauritius. *British Medical Journal*, 1995, **311**:1255–1259.

25. Hypertension Prevention Trial Research Group. The hypertension prevention trial: three-year effects of dietary change on blood pressure. *Archives of Internal Medicine*, 1990, **150**:153–162.

26. **Hall SM et al.** Weight gain prevention and smoking cessation: cautionary findings. *American Journal of Public Health*, 1992, **82**:799–803.

27. **King AC.** Community intervention for promotion of physical activity and fitness. *Exercise and Sport Sciences Reviews*, 1991, **19**:211–259.

28. **Booth M et al.** Effects of a national mass-media campaign on physical activity participation. *Health Promotion International*, 1992, **7**:241–247.

29. **Owen N et al.** Serial mass-media campaigns to promote physical activity: reinforcing or redundant. *American Journal of Public Health*, 1995, **85**:244–248.

30. **Tverdal A.** Hoyde, vekt og kroppsmasseindeks for menn og kvinner i alderen 40–42 år. [Height, weight and body mass index for men and women aged 40–42 years.] *Tidsskrift for den Norske Laegeforening*, 1996, **116**:2152–2156.

31. **Jeffery RW.** Public health approaches to the management of obesity. In: Brownell KD, Fairburn CG, eds. *Eating disorders and obesity: a comprehensive handbook*. London, Guilford Press, 1995:558–563.

32. **Gill TP.** Key issues in the prevention of obesity. *British Medical Bulletin*, 1997, **53**:359–388.

33. **Borland R, Owen N.** Regulatory innovations, behaviour and health: implications of research on workplace smoking bans. *International Reviews of Health Psychology*, 1994, **3**:167–185.

34. **Reynolds C.** Legislation and the new public health: introduction. *Community Health Studies*, 1989, **13**:397–402.

35. **LeFebvre CR, Flora JA.** Social marketing and public health intervention. *Health Education Quarterly*, 1988, **15**:219–315.

36. **Forte JG.** Salt and blood pressure: a community trial. *Journal of Human Hypertension*, 1989, **3**:179–184.

37. **Clancey-Hepburn K, Hickey A, Neville G.** Children's behaviour responses to TV food advertisements. *Journal of Nutrition Education*, 1974, **6**:93–96.

38. **Taras HL et al.** Television's influence on children's diet and physical activity. *Journal of Developmental and Behavioral Pediatrics*, 1989, **10**:176–180.

39. **Woodward DR et al.** Does television affect teenagers' diet? *Proceedings of the Nutrition Society of Australia*, 1992, **17**:48.

40. **Robinson TN, Killen JD.** Ethnic and gender differences in the relationships between television viewing and obesity, physical activity and dietary fat intake. *Journal of Health Education*, 1995, **26**(Suppl.):91–98.

41. Massachusetts Medical Society Committee on Nutrition. Fast food fare: consumer guidelines. *New England Journal of Medicine*, 1990, **321**:752–755.

42. Allied Dunbar, Health Education Authority, Sports Council. *Allied Dunbar National Fitness Survey: a summary of the major findings and message from the Allied Dunbar National Fitness Survey*. London, Health Education Authority and Sports Council, 1992.

43. **Moor BJ et al.** Neighbourhood safety, child care and high cost of fruits and vegetables identified as barriers to increased activity and healthy eating and linked to overweight and income. *FASEB Journal*, 1996, **10**(3):A562.

10. Prevention and management of overweight and obesity in at-risk individuals: an integrated health-care services approach in community settings

10.1 Introduction

This section deals with programmes intended for individuals and groups already overweight or obese, or at particularly high risk of obesity and its comorbidities. Particular emphasis is placed on an integrated health care services approach in community settings. It should be noted that:

- Effective weight management for individuals and groups at risk of developing obesity involves the whole range of long-term strategies mentioned in section 8.2, namely prevention, weight maintenance, management of comorbidities and weight loss.

- No long-term trials have been conducted on the effectiveness of obesity prevention *per se* through health-care services or in community settings. Preliminary evidence suggests that low-intensity educational and incentive programmes aimed directly at preventing weight gain in adults can have a positive impact on body weight.

- An effective weight-management protocol consists of the following five main stages: recruitment and referral; comprehensive health assessment; goal-setting; selection and implementation of an appropriate management scheme; and monitoring and evaluation.

- A personal support scheme for the overweight and obese patient, including family involvement and trained personnel, can considerably improve the outcome in terms of weight loss and weight maintenance. Well run self-help groups also offer a useful and inexpensive form of continuing support. Commercial weight-loss organizations can be of use in weight management provided that they follow a code of practice covering fees, the training of counsellors and the promotion of services.

- A number of well established and properly evaluated treatments are available for obesity, including dietary management, physical activity, behaviour modification, drug therapy and gastric surgery.

- Modest energy-deficit diets appear to be more effective and acceptable than severe energy deficits in achieving and maintaining weight loss. The effectiveness of dietary therapy is greatly improved if exercise and behaviour modification are included in an individually tailored plan. Further evaluation of current lifestyle strategies and the combined therapies is required to determine their usefulness in achieving long-term weight loss.

- Drug treatment may be appropriate for high-risk obese patients for whom changes in lifestyle alone have been unsuccessful in reducing weight. Weight-management drugs should be used only under medical supervision so that the risks associated with drug treatment can be balanced against those of persisting obesity. Long-term administration, as part of a management strategy tailored to the individual, would appear to be the most logical and effective way of using weight-management drugs. However, data on the risk–benefit ratio of the long-term use of these drugs are still lacking.

- Gastric surgery is considered to be the most effective way of reducing weight and maintaining weight loss in severely obese patients.

- The objectives of weight-management strategies for children differ from those for adults because consideration needs to be given to the physical and intellectual development of the child. In contrast to adult treatment, which may be aimed at weight loss, child treatment is aimed at preventing weight gain.

- Three strategies for the treatment of obese children are available: reduction of energy intake, increased physical activity and reduction of inactivity. Primary health-care services, families and schools are all useful and appropriate settings for the prevention and treatment of obesity in children.

10.2 Management strategies for at-risk individuals and groups

The effective management of individuals and groups who are obese, or who are at particular risk of becoming so, demands health professionals with expertise in obesity management. Such professionals require knowledge, skills and attitudes appropriate to obesity management, and need to use the whole range of approaches shown in Fig. 8.1, p. 157, namely: prevention of weight gain, promotion of weight maintenance, management of obesity comorbidities and promotion of weight loss.

10.2.1 Prevention of weight gain

Prevention is probably the most effective, but currently underutilized, approach to weight management. It was suggested in section 8 that prevention can be divided into three levels, two of which are concerned with those who are at high risk of weight gain and its consequences, namely:

- *Selective prevention* — directed at high-risk individuals and groups.

- *Targeted prevention* — directed at those with existing weight problems and those at high risk of diseases associated with overweight.

Weight-management programmes can therefore be initiated to target those high-risk individuals and subgroups of the population identified in section 7.

As pointed out in section 8, there is an urgent need for intervention studies specifically aimed at preventing weight gain in adults. So far, the results of only two such studies have been reported. The first was a small-scale trial in a relatively select group[1] of normal-weight individuals to determine whether a low-impact intervention involving an educational programme (four nutrition education sessions and a monthly weight-control information newsletter) and a financial incentive could reduce weight gain. After 1 year, those in the treated group had lost about 1 kg in weight, while the weights of those in the control group remained unchanged (*1*). Analysis of the results showed that the greatest impact was among men, individuals over the age of 50, non-smokers and those with little prior experience of formal weight-loss services. The second report describes the first-year results of the Pound of Prevention (POP) study, an ongoing continuation of the first study that adopts a similar approach but applies it to a larger population (more than 1000 participants) over a longer period (*2*). Among men and high-income women, early trends in combating weight gain were encouraging and, if sustained over 3 years, should produce a positive outcome. However, trends in the low-income group were negative at 1 year. Further follow-up will reveal whether the low-intensity educational strategy being tested is effective in reducing the rate of weight gain in the groups being studied, and the study may help to identify behavioural correlates of weight gain that could provide guidance for further research on this important topic.

Prevention at the workplace

In recent years, health education interventions at workplaces have been a popular method of targeting high-risk individuals and groups, but most studies have been of short duration. Longer-term interventions aimed at high-risk individuals, such as the 6-year WHO European Collaborative Trial of Multifactorial Prevention of Coronary Heart Disease (*3*), in which some workers in factories underwent risk-factor screening (serum cholesterol, blood pressure, smoking) and medical follow-up, proved to be ineffective in lowering BMI. In the

---

[1] Recruited among individuals who had participated in a risk-factor screening programme.

USA, a 2-year study of cigarette smoking and obesity found no differences in the mean BMI or any change in BMI at workplaces that offered weight-loss classes (on four occasions) compared with those that did not (*4*).

Prevention through health care services
To date, there have been no long-term trials on the effectiveness of obesity prevention *per se* through health-care services (see section 8). However, in one practice in the United Kingdom, the provision of healthy eating advice to pregnant women and their children restricted the prevalence of obesity to only 2% compared with levels closer to 8% in subjects who were not offered advice (*5*). On a larger scale, two controlled screening and intervention programmes aimed at reducing CHD risk factors through instruction and support from nurses in general practice have been evaluated recently. Both the OXCHECK Study (*6*) and the Family Heart Study (*7*) were able to demonstrate small but significant differences in weight of 0.5–1.5% between intervention and control groups after only 1 year. The intervention was aimed at altering diet quality rather than serving as a specific obesity-management scheme.

10.2.2 Weight maintenance

Long-term weight maintenance is not only relevant to those who have recently lost weight, but is also an important element of all weight-management programmes. Rössner (*8*) has highlighted this issue by recognizing that the natural trend of BMI in most developed countries is to increase with age. A body weight kept constant over a decade as a result of a weight-management programme therefore represents a successful outcome, and is a particularly valuable achievement in those patients who have family histories of obesity and/or its medical complications, and who are particularly prone to weight gain and obesity. Weight maintenance is shown in Fig. 10.1 as one of a range of indicators of success in obesity-management programmes. Weight maintenance and minor or modest weight loss are more likely to be achieved than weight normalization.

10.2.3 Management of obesity comorbidities

The management of obesity comorbidities can improve health outcomes regardless of whether or not substantial weight loss is achieved (*9, 10*). As highlighted in section 4, such comorbidities range from chronic debilitating, though not life-threatening, conditions to severe health risks associated with hyperlipidaemia and hypertension. Appropriate targets relating to the management of obesity comorbidities are suggested in Table 10.1.

Figure 10.1
Possible indicators of success in obesity-management programmes[a]

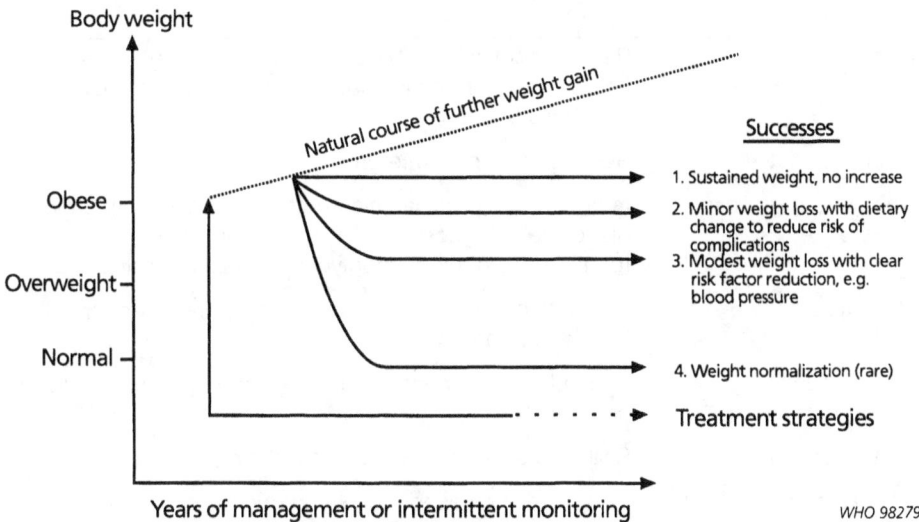

Weight maintenance or minor weight loss are successful outcomes of programmes aimed at controlling obesity when otherwise (without intervention) weight gain would occur.

[a] Adapted from reference 8 with the permission of the publisher and author.

10.2.4 *Weight loss*

The benefits of modest, intentional weight loss have been described in section 5. Doctors and their patients need to recognize that moderate but sustained weight loss in the range 5–15% of initial weight is medically highly advantageous if long-lasting (9, 11). Substantial improvements in obesity comorbidities result, particularly in hypertension and in blood glucose and plasma lipid levels.

However, a return to the so-called "ideal body weight" has for too long been considered by the medical profession to be both a possible and a mandatory target for obese people. This misconception has been transmitted to the public, and has been reinforced by the promotion by the mass media of slenderness as the ideal body image. As a result, there is now considerable pressure on the overweight individual to return to his/her ideal, often at the lower end of the normal (18.5–25) BMI range.

Returning to an ideal body weight is not an appropriate goal for the following reasons:

• Weight gain is a health risk, and this risk is independent of the actual level of BMI (12).

Table 10.1

Appropriate targets for the management of obesity and comorbidities

Condition	Appropriate target[a]
Fatness	Reduce body weight by 5–15% (smaller weight loss is also acceptable if abdominal fat loss is sufficient to provide metabolic benefit)
Abdominal fat	Reduce waist circumference
NIDDM and glucose intolerance	Improvement in glycaemic control, i.e. fall in fasting blood glucose and glycosylated haemoglobin levels, and reduced use of oral hypoglycaemic agents and/or insulin
Hypertension	Fall in blood pressure and reduction in the need for hypotensive agents
Dyslipidaemia	Defined improvements in LDL, fasting triglycerides, HDL cholesterol
Sleep apnoea	Reduced sleep apnoea, improved lung function
Arthritis and back pain	Pain relief, increased mobility; reduced need for drug therapy
Reproductive dysfunction	Improved reproductive function with regular menstruation
Poor psychosocial functioning	Improved quality of life; reduced anxiety; reduced depression; improved social interaction
Tiredness, sweating, breathlessness etc.	Resolution or reduction of severity
Exercise intolerance	Improved exercise tolerance; reduced breathlessness

[a] Quantitative estimates of magnitude of change in target value may vary for specific populations.

- Substantial benefit, e.g. a 25% decline in mortality, can accrue from weight losses of 5–10 kg in 1 year (*10*).

- Physiological responses limit weight loss, so that it is unusual to return to normal weight unless patients are very persistent and effective in monitoring and controlling their drive to eat. Severe dietary restrictions are unhealthy and may precipitate eating disorders in some circumstances (*13*).

- Repeated failures to achieve and sustain substantial weight loss may increase a patient's depression and lack of self-esteem and may result in further weight gain.

- Long-term health depends on limiting weight gain over time.

- Clinical trials show that most patients are unable to continue losing weight for longer than 12–16 weeks (4–8 kg loss) and that weight loss does not continue after 6 months (*14*). Patients are seldom applauded or rewarded for achieving this modest loss, even though it requires prolonged hard work and brings major health benefits.

10.3 A health-care services approach to the new concept of weight management

In response to the failure of current obesity-management practices to deal effectively with the problem of obesity, several expert working groups have recently examined how the management of obesity in health-care services could be improved.

A coordinated approach to obesity management in line with the strategies outlined in section 9 is required. A primary goal of long-term weight maintenance should be combined with appropriate treatment for modest weight loss and the management of comorbidities in overweight patients. Prevention of weight gain in those individuals who are at risk of becoming obese in the future is also crucial (*15–17*).

It is anticipated that each country will need to modify and develop the guidelines according to its own particular needs and health care structures. However, the basic principles of an effective weight-management protocol remain the same and involve the following five main stages:

— recruitment and referral;
— comprehensive health assessment;
— goal-setting;
— selection and implementation of an appropriate management scheme;
— monitoring and evaluation.

10.3.1 *Recruitment and referral*

Recruiting at-risk groups and individuals is the first step in an effective weight-management protocol. The three main methods of recruitment and referral are as follows:

- *Public awareness campaigns* highlighting the dangers of excess weight associated with high BMI and/or waist circumference, e.g. through school health services, insurance agencies and employers.

- *Opportunistic screening* of patients who present for other conditions, e.g. infections, trauma or other intercurrent illness.

- *Public health screening* incorporated into other health service activities and programmes, e.g. immunization, mother and infant welfare clinics, and screening programmes for tuberculosis, infestations and cancer of breast and cervix.

10.3.2 *Comprehensive health assessment*

The development of an effective weight-management strategy depends on a comprehensive analysis of the individual's degree of obesity, his or her associated risks, coexisting illnesses, social and personal situation, and a history of those problems and precipitating factors that led to weight gain. The components of such an analysis might include those outlined below.

Personal weight history
Patients can be categorized according to a simple scheme by means of a series of standardized questions based on, e.g. current BMI; current state of energy balance (as indicated by actual weight kinetics, i.e. weight gain, loss or stability); weight at specific ages; age of onset of weight gain; peak weight; lowest weight maintained for one or more years; and number of weight-loss attempts.

The environmental circumstances and the life events that have had a temporal relationship to weight gain or regain can be useful in developing behavioural strategies for altering lifestyles.

Physical activity
Simple questionnaires are now available that allow an assessment to be made of levels of occupational and recreational activity (*18*).

Dietary patterns
Information on habitual food intake, meal patterns and reasons for eating can be obtained from a dietary record or brief interview. Patients with eating disorders should be identified by means of questionnaires or interviews, and appropriate strategies should be included in the management plan to deal with them.

Recommended methods of dietary assessment tend to be appropriate only for epidemiological research and not for use in a clinical setting (*19*). Recording bias, particularly under-reporting by obese subjects, is a problem. Generally, food diaries have been adapted to include behavioural questions and quantitative scales for describing patients' feelings, but no single accepted format is widely used (*20*).

Assessment of health indicators and risk factors
The following health indicators and risk factors should be assessed:

- *Fat distribution.* Individuals at high risk due to abdominal fat distribution can be identified by measuring waist circumference or waist: hip ratio (section 2).

- *Smoking.* Smoking is particularly important because some patients use tobacco as a means of limiting weight gain despite the major risks associated with the tobacco use (*21*).

- *Drug use.* Several drugs used to treat medical conditions promote weight gain (Table 7.6).

- *Family history.* A family history of certain diseases (CVD, NIDDM, hyperlipidaemia or hypertension) increases the risk that obese individuals or those gaining weight are likely to develop these complications.

Psychosocial and behavioural assessment

It is important to assess and understand the psychological and social characteristics of the individual (*22, 23*) as these can be important in determining the best weight-management strategy.

A psychosocial assessment might include the determination of occupational circumstances, the structure of the nuclear family and the degree of family support, the reasons why the patient wishes to lose weight, and the presence of mood disturbances. There is a need for validated questionnaires, e.g. on depression, anxiety, eating behaviour, etc., that are appropriate to the culture concerned.

Medical examination

A routine medical examination should include physical examination, measurement of blood pressure, and anthropometry, which usually includes, in addition to BMI, waist circumference, hip circumference and measurement of several skinfold thicknesses as an approximate measure of fat stores. Waist circumference is a good indicator of risk associated with the complications of obesity (e.g. hypertension) and is easy to measure.

Laboratory tests

Where resources are available, the health assessment might include the analysis of blood and urine for metabolites indicative of disease risk, e.g. plasma glucose and blood lipids. Some tests carried out routinely in overweight and obese patients (e.g. hormone levels for rare abnormalities) are considered to be an unwise use of resources.

10.3.3 Setting appropriate targets

The information gained from the comprehensive health assessment should enable doctor and patient to agree on a realistic and appropriate goal. This is essential in developing a suitable management plan for patients and groups, and for assessing progress and success.

The management goal should not be chosen solely on the basis of BMI, but should also take into account the presence of other risk factors and social and personal circumstances. This is illustrated in Fig. 10.2, which presents an algorithm for a systematic approach to obesity management through health care services. Experience has shown that clearly defined practical guidelines for the general public and for health professionals are needed to minimize resistance to, and confusion about, setting appropriate weight goals (24).

The American Obesity Association (17), a Scottish group (16), and a recent report of a subgroup of the International Obesity Task Force[1] all support a strategy for setting appropriate management goals based on the following values of BMI (special values of cut-offs (see Table 2.1) for ethnic subgroups may need to be selected):

- *BMI 25–29.9.* Where there are no risk factors such as increased waist circumference, the emphasis should be on weight stability. Where comorbidities are present, risk management through changes in diet, exercise and lifestyle is necessary. Weight-loss goals should be introduced if the health risks are not substantially reduced within a few months.

- *BMI ≥30.* This is associated with a much higher risk of morbidity, so that long-term weight management with some preliminary weight loss is advisable. When health risks are extremely high (e.g. BMI >40), and conventional treatment has failed to reduce them appropriately, patients should be referred to a specialized service so that the need for surgery can be properly evaluated.

10.3.4 *Selection and implementation of appropriate management strategies*

Different strategies will be required to meet the objectives of the different elements of weight management.

For *weight maintenance*, and for *prevention of weight gain* in at-risk individuals, healthier eating and a more active lifestyle are necessary. For *weight loss*, or to decrease body fat, a temporary negative energy (or fat) balance must be created so that fat stores can be used to meet energy demands. This means either reducing intake or increasing energy expenditure or both. *Management of comorbid conditions* may require special attention to be paid to specific dietary features, e.g. salt intake in hypertensive patients.

---

[1] Deslypere JP, ed. *The management of obesity through health care services*, 1996. Background paper prepared by Primary Health Care–Specialist Interface subgroup of the International Obesity Task Force.

Figure 10.2

A systematic approach to obesity management based on BMI and other risk factors

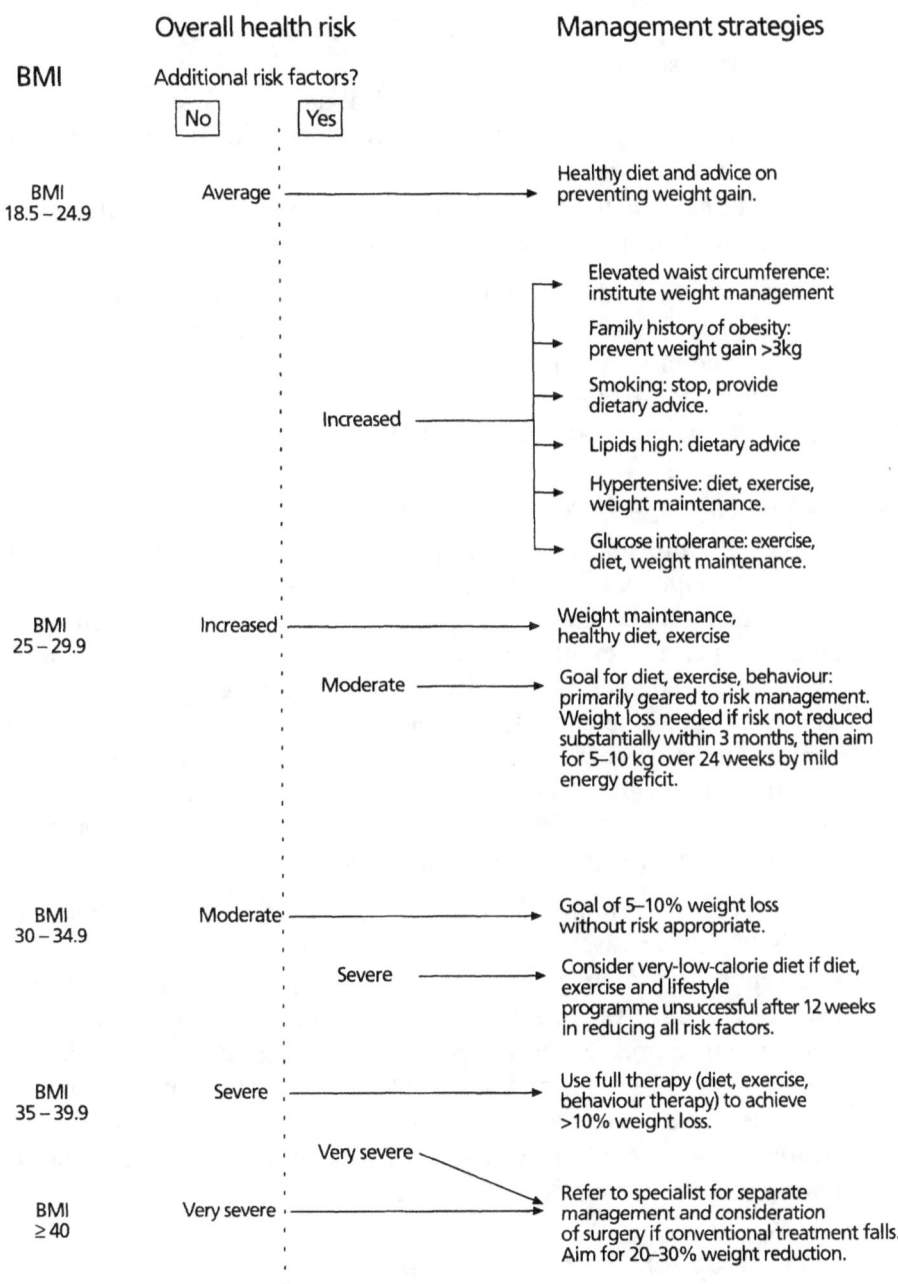

Assess overall health risk from BMI and other risk factors, e.g. waist circumference

Overall health risk — Management strategies

BMI — Additional risk factors? No / Yes

BMI 18.5 – 24.9 — Average — Healthy diet and advice on preventing weight gain.

Increased:
- Elevated waist circumference: institute weight management
- Family history of obesity: prevent weight gain >3kg
- Smoking: stop, provide dietary advice.
- Lipids high: dietary advice
- Hypertensive: diet, exercise, weight maintenance.
- Glucose intolerance: exercise, diet, weight maintenance.

BMI 25 – 29.9 — Increased — Weight maintenance, healthy diet, exercise

Moderate — Goal for diet, exercise, behaviour: primarily geared to risk management. Weight loss needed if risk not reduced substantially within 3 months, then aim for 5–10 kg over 24 weeks by mild energy deficit.

BMI 30 – 34.9 — Moderate — Goal of 5–10% weight loss without risk appropriate.

Severe — Consider very-low-calorie diet if diet, exercise and lifestyle programme unsuccessful after 12 weeks in reducing all risk factors.

BMI 35 – 39.9 — Severe — Use full therapy (diet, exercise, behaviour therapy) to achieve >10% weight loss.

Very severe

BMI ≥ 40 — Very severe — Refer to specialist for separate management and consideration of surgery if conventional treatment falls. Aim for 20–30% weight reduction.

WHO 98272

207

The development of successful weight-management schemes requires patient cooperation and motivation and involves five linked components:

— a personal support scheme that includes specially trained personnel and, if possible and appropriate, family involvement;
— dietary assessment followed by individually tailored advice;
— analysis and modification of physical activity patterns;
— behavioural advice that links environmental and psychosocial factors to the changes needed in diet and physical activity;
— additional treatments may also be indicated depending on the degree of overweight and the presence of comorbidities.

The various methods of treatment available for obesity are outlined in section 10.5. The suitability of any particular treatment will depend on BMI, on the targets that have been set, and on the clinical characteristics of the patients as determined in the assessment stage. A combination of several treatments is usually advisable.

10.3.5 *Monitoring, rewards and evaluation*

Regular monitoring of patients' progress is probably one of the most important aspects of the weight-management process; it should not cease when patients have reached agreed goals but should form part of continuing care. Regular review allows weight-management progress to be supported, medical conditions to be monitored, and problems to be dealt with at the earliest possible opportunity. It is important that achievements in weight maintenance or weight loss (no matter how small) are recognized, and a programme of rewards for achieving set goals is often useful. Such rewards should be non-food-based and agreed with a patient at an early stage of management.

An equally important aspect of any obesity-management approach within health care systems is the constant evaluation of the efficacy of different weight-management strategies. Systems for auditing the efficacy of current practices should be integrated into the health care delivery structures. Such an approach requires long-term follow-up of patients and groups recruited into different weight-management schemes. For example, an indication of whether a weight-maintenance strategy is successful or not could be gained by considering whether one or more of the criteria presented in Table 10.2 have been met.

10.4 **Patient support in obesity treatment**

There is considerable evidence to suggest that patient support by health professionals, peers and family members can notably increase successful weight loss and weight maintenance (25–27).

Table 10.2
Potential criteria for evaluating weight-maintenance strategy

- Maintenance of a stable weight over time (even if BMI is not reduced to within the normal range)
- Reduction in the number of obese people who develop obesity-related comorbidities
- Increase in the number of obese people who are successful in attaining and maintaining modest weight losses
- Reduction in the number of individuals who gain even a small amount of weight over a specified period
- Low withdrawal rates
- Low relapse rates
- Improvement in risk factors and comorbidities

10.4.1 *Support within the health-care service*

Evaluation of weight-management programmes within health-care settings suggests that (*28*):

- Specially trained health personnel (e.g. nurses, dietitians, trained lay persons) produce better results than untrained staff involved in routine medical management.

- Visits at short intervals, rather than monthly or at longer intervals, are of greater value.

- With most patients, better responses are achieved in a group setting.

Thus trained personnel who have frequent contact with patients, preferably as part of a support group, are recommended. In addition, efforts should be made to prevent guilt feelings associated with the obese state.

10.4.2 *Involvement of family*

A number of studies have shown that the body weight and attitudes of a patient's spouse can have a major impact on the amount of weight lost and on success in weight maintenance. Black & Threlfall (*29*) found that overweight patients with normal-weight partners lost significantly more weight than those with overweight partners. They also noted that success was greater in those patients whose partners had also lost weight (even though they were not included in the programme), suggesting that recommended changes were being actively supported by the spouse. Similarly, Pratt found that drop-out rates were reduced when the patient's spouse was included in a weight-control programme (*30*).

Additional evidence for the important role of family support in successful weight management is provided by the work of Epstein and colleagues (*31*) on the treatment of childhood obesity.

10.4.3 *Self-help and support groups*

In recent years there has been a large increase in the number of self-help and support groups. These range from national organizations such as Overeaters Anonymous (OA) in the USA and Anonymous Fighters Against Obesity (ALCO) in Argentina, Chile, Paraguay, Spain and Uruguay, to smaller workplace, neighbourhood and community-organized self-help groups. These groups generally consist of people with weight or eating problems, and operate at little or no cost and without professional intervention. They all offer considerable social support but vary in their philosophy. Unfortunately, although such groups are immensely popular, there has been no objective assessment of their value in weight management. However, well run self-help groups are a useful and inexpensive form of continuing group support; they encourage long-term participation and can be a useful adjunct to professional care.

Advocacy groups for overweight and obese persons, such as the Size Acceptance Network in the USA, serve a different function from self-help groups, aiming to reduce the stigma and social difficulties that obese patients suffer. Recently, a patient support and advocacy group called EUROBESITAS has been established to lobby for the rights of obese patients in Europe.

10.4.4 *Commercial weight-loss organizations*

Numerous commercial organizations offer a mixture of instruction, guidance and support in weight loss. They are usually not run by health professionals, although they may be based on material produced by them and on advice from professional consultants. All such organizations rely on counsellors (who vary in their level of training) to provide services to individual clients for a fee. Regular sessions cover a wide variety of subjects ranging from specific information on dieting, nutrition and physical activity, to techniques for changing behaviour. The cost of such programmes varies enormously, from a nominal fee paid at each session to very large sums paid on joining to purchase special dietary supplements and prepackaged foods that form part of the programme.

There is some concern about the regulation of commercial weight-loss organizations. There is a risk of financial exploitation, and counsellors may be completely untrained. Attempts to evaluate the effectiveness of commercial programmes have resulted in few objective assessments because of problems of confidentiality, drop-out rates and lack of interest among the organizations themselves (*32*). The US Food and Nutrition Board Committee has suggested that there is a need for guidelines on voluntary accreditation within the commercial weight-loss industry (*15*). The misleading marketing of weight-loss programmes has often been a cause of complaints to consumer organizations.

Nevertheless, many well run programmes provide the support and interest needed for long-term involvement in weight management that cannot be provided by health professionals. Commercial weight-loss organizations should therefore be required to comply with a code of practice in relation to fees, training of counsellors and promotion of their services. They should also report the outcomes of their programmes. Health professionals may consider the judicious use of such organizations in obesity management after assessing their merit, using the criteria suggested by the Scottish Intercollegiate Guidelines Network (Annex 1).

10.5 Treatment of obesity

A wide variety of treatments for obesity are available, including dietary management, physical activity, behaviour modification, pharmacological treatment and surgery. However, there is a need to control the promotion of dangerous and deliberately deceptive approaches to weight loss or control, such as special weight-loss aids, equipment, "miracle cures", and certain drugs and treatments often offered through unlicensed weight-loss centres.

10.5.1 *Dietary management*

The education of overweight patients about foods and eating habits that facilitate weight control is an essential component of all weight-management strategies. Dietary intake and patterns should be assessed to identify areas requiring special attention such as nutritional adequacy, meal size, meal frequency and meal timing.

Dietary restriction represents the most conventional "treatment" for overweight and obesity. It usually induces weight loss in the short term, but its poor long-term effectiveness, especially when used in isolation, is widely recognized (*33*). Diets based on healthy eating principles, including the individualized modest energy-deficit diet and the *ad libitum* low-fat diet, appear to have a better long-term outcome. Further randomized, controlled, long-term dietary intervention studies are needed to identify the optimal diet for the treatment of obesity (i.e. weight loss, weight maintenance and management of comorbidities).

Individualized modest energy-deficit diets

This dietary scheme is based on inducing an energy deficit that patients can sustain over the long term. A deficit of 500–600 kcal$_{th}$/day (2092–2510 kJ/day) is usually well tolerated. When used correctly, this approach has resulted in larger weight losses over time than attempting more severe energy restriction (*34*).

The specific energy intake prescribed to patients is based on an estimate of their initial maintenance requirement minus the agreed deficit. Maintenance estimates should be calculated from the equations of Lean & James (*35*), based on body weight and age, rather than from self-reported dietary intakes since these are notoriously unreliable when obtained from obese subjects (*36*). After subtracting the deficit, the energy prescription can be translated into a dietary plan using a food exchange table based on healthy eating principles, i.e. approximately 20–30% or less energy as fat, 15% as protein, and 55–60% or more as carbohydrate (primarily complex carbohydrates). The assessment of current dietary patterns should be used to construct and educate the patient to follow a dietary plan appropriate to his or her circumstances. The prescribed energy level of such plans should generally not be lower than 1200 kcal$_{th}$/day (5021 kJ/day).

Low-fat, high-carbohydrate diets

The main argument in favour of low-fat diets is their beneficial effect on CVD risk factors (*37*). However, such diets have also been shown to cause weight loss proportional to pretreatment weight, and to the long-term reduction in dietary fat content. Astrup et al. (*38*), for example, found that a reduction of 10% in fat energy could produce an average 5-kg weight loss in obese subjects, although a number of other studies have failed to give the same result.

After major weight loss, an *ad libitum* low-fat high-carbohydrate diet programme has been shown to be superior to calorie-counting in maintaining weight loss 2 years later (*39*). Replacing a proportion of the fat by protein instead of carbohydrate may further increase the weight loss.

Severe/moderate energy-deficit diets

The standard practice in many lay and commercial systems for slimming is for the patient to be prescribed a standard energy intake, normally 1000–1200 kcal$_{th}$/day (4184–5021 kJ/day). These intakes are usually selected by dietitians or doctors in accordance with nutritional guidelines for healthy people and are prescribed, unchanged, to large numbers of adults. However, not all patients have the same energy requirements, and the magnitude of the energy deficit imposed by the diet will be greater with higher energy requirements. Furthermore, energy intake at this level is usually associated with a deficient intake of several nutrients.

Based on published studies, diets providing fewer than 1200 kcal$_{th}$ (4184 kJ) induce up to 15% weight loss over 10–20 weeks (40) but, without a maintenance programme, most of the weight lost is regained (41). Patients are rarely assessed for longer than a year, and most of the trials that induce this rate of weight loss have, in fact, combined behaviour modification with the dietary regimen. Drop-out rates tend to be high, although major improvements in compliance and continuing involvement in weight management can be made if associated support systems are established to cope with patients' needs.

Very-low-calorie diets
Very-low-calorie diets (VLCDs) can induce rapid weight loss over a 3-month period but do not seem particularly conducive to long-term weight maintenance (42, 43). They should usually be reserved for achieving rapid short-term weight loss on medical grounds (e.g. before surgery) in patients with a BMI >30. The use of VLCDs by individuals without medical supervision is unwise and should not be recommended.

Concerns over loss of body protein/lean tissues with traditional VLCDs highlighted the need for a minimum energy level and the proper formulation of such diets. Nowadays, VLCDs usually provide a ketogenic (high-protein, high-fat, low-carbohydrate) diet with an acceptable minimum energy level of 800 kcal$_{th}$/day (3347 kJ/day) in the form of protein-, mineral- and vitamin-enriched meals or drinks. Research has shown that VLCDs with energy levels of less than 800 kcal$_{th}$/day (3347 kJ/day) do not produce greater weight loss, and are less well accepted, than diets providing this energy level (44).

10.5.2 *Physical activity and exercise*

The combination of exercise and diet is more effective than either method alone in promoting fat loss (45). Exercise also limits the proportion of lean tissue lost in slimming regimens (46) and limits weight regain (45, 47), while physical activity may favourably affect body fat distribution (48).

Physical activity has numerous beneficial effects regardless of BMI and age. Individuals who engage in moderate or vigorous exercise at

Table 10.3
Suggested mechanisms linking exercise with the success of weight maintenance[a]

Increased energy expenditure
Better aerobic fitness
Improved body composition:
fat loss
preservation of lean body mass
reduction of visceral fat depot
Increased capacity for fat mobilization and oxidation
Control of food intake:
short-term reduction of appetite
reduction of fat intake
Stimulation of thermogenic response:
resting metabolic rate
diet-induced thermogenesis
Change in muscle morphology and biochemical capacity
Increased insulin sensitivity
Improved plasma lipid and lipoprotein profile
Reduced blood pressure
Positive psychological effects

[a] Reproduced from reference *50* with the permission of the publisher. Copyright John Wiley & Sons Ltd.

least once a week are less likely to have NIDDM or CVD, hip fractures and mental illness, and have lower mortality rates than those who are least active. Integrated exercise schemes consistently show the beneficial effects of physical activity and exercise on both physiological and psychological well-being (*48, 49*).

Table 10.3 summarizes the possible mechanisms whereby exercise can improve the success of weight maintenance.

Achieving appropriate levels of physical activity
Evidence now suggests that the activity required to maintain and lose weight, and to gain physiological and psychological health benefits, may not have to be as vigorous as was previously believed (*48, 51*). Indeed, the US Surgeon General's report (*48*) stressed that low-intensity, prolonged physical activity, such as purposeful walking for 30–60 minutes almost every day, can substantially increase energy expenditure, thus reducing body weight and fat.

Physical activity strategies should aim at encouraging higher levels of low-intensity activity and reducing the amount of leisure time spent in sedentary pursuits. The main goal is to convert inactive children and adults to a pattern of "active living". Two general schemes can be envisaged for promoting physical activity:

- *Measures to increase modest daily exercise*, as in walking or cycling, where the energy expended amounts to about an extra 60–200 kcal$_{th}$/h (125.5–251 kJ/h) depending on the intensity of the exercise. In sedentary overweight and obese patients, an extra 3 hours daily of any activity involving standing rather than sitting increases the 24-hour energy expenditure from 40% to more than 75% above the BMR (*52*).

- *Physiological fitness training with moderate/vigorous exercise*, usually involving group-supervised exercise sessions of 45–60 minutes each three times a week. Extensive studies show that these regimens have very substantial benefits but are difficult to sustain in obese patients.

More intensive degrees of exercise need to be considered on an individual basis in overweight and obese patients. Breathlessness and musculoskeletal problems are common in the obese, and will prevent them from sustaining exercise that uses a substantial amount of energy.

Improving compliance
Analysis of randomized trials of public involvement in physical activity programmes (*53*) has indicated that compliance is improved by:

— home-based activities rather than structured programmes in a special facility or centre;
— encouragement by frequent professional contact either by telephone or home visit;
— social support, particularly from family members (*16*);
— informal and unsupervised exercise;
— low/moderate-intensity exercise;
— promoting walking as a form of exercise;
— taking exercise from time to time during the day rather than in a single burst of continuous activity (*48*).

On this basis, additional walking or other modest exercise may prove most conducive to maintaining compliance in overweight and obese patients. The first three items in the list are also relevant to improved dietary compliance.

10.5.3 Behaviour modification

The primary goal of behavioural treatment is the improvement of eating habits (i.e. what to eat, where to eat, when to eat, how to eat) and levels of physical activity. Behavioural treatment is considered to be an essential component of any adequate obesity-treatment programme (*54*).

Method of treatment
Behavioural treatment has a number of core features:

- *Self-monitoring*: the detailed, daily recording of food intake and the circumstances in which it occurs provides the essential information needed for selecting and implementing intervention strategies. It also forms part of the behaviour modification process, through evaluation of progress, and identification of personal and environmental influences that regulate eating and physical activity.

- *Stimulus control*: limiting exposure to cues that prompt overeating. For example, patients are instructed to separate eating from other activities so that they remain fully aware of their actions.

- *Emphasis on improved nutrition*: rigid dieting is discouraged in favour of balanced and flexible food choices.

- *Cognitive restructuring*: a method of identifying and modifying dysfunctional thoughts and attitudes about weight regulation.

- *Study of interpersonal relationships*: assists in coping with specific triggers for overeating and in increasing social support for weight control.

- *Relapse prevention*: a continuing process designed to promote the maintenance of treatment-induced weight loss.

Evaluation of treatment outcome
Behavioural treatment has been more intensively researched, and its effects more thoroughly documented, than any other obesity intervention. It is effective in changing behaviour in the short term and consistently produces significant weight loss in patients with mild to moderate obesity. In the long term, however, results are not encouraging, virtually all adult patients returning to their pretreatment baseline within 5 years (44). Long-term outcomes in children, by contrast, are more promising (55); they indicate that behavioural changes resulting from family-based therapy last 10 years or more. Further research is needed on ways of increasing the effectiveness of behavioural techniques.

Limitations of behavioural treatment
It is thought that behavioural treatment is ineffective in the long term because patients fail to follow the self-regulatory strategies that they learn in treatment. Some investigators have therefore stressed the need for lifelong treatment; obesity is a chronic condition and treatments, whether behavioural, dietary or pharmacological, do not work when they are not used (54).

Other benefits of behavioural treatment
Despite its limitations in producing long-term weight loss, behavioural treatment is of value in modifying behaviours linked to adverse health effects and psychological distress, without necessarily causing weight loss in obese individuals. It can also promote behaviours that directly affect health, such as reducing fat intake and increasing physical activity, although there are also problems in sustaining them in the long term. Finally, behavioural treatment can be used to help obese patients to become more assertive in coping with the adverse social consequences of being overweight, to enhance their self-esteem, and to reduce their dissatisfaction with their body image regardless of their lack of success in losing weight (56).

10.5.4 *Drug treatment*

The information presented here was up to date at the time of writing, but drug treatment of obesity is constantly changing.

Drug treatment of obesity has often been seen as controversial, largely because of failure to understand how it should be used. However, it has been re-evaluated in recent years and the concept of long-term drug treatment has emerged as an adjunct to other weight-loss therapies and as a way of helping to maintain body weight over time (57).

Due to the paucity of data, no particular strategy or drug can yet be recommended for routine use. However, the availability of new evidence of the long-term efficacy and safety of several drugs currently awaiting approval is likely to change the situation. When the pharmacological treatment of obese patients is prescribed in the future, it will be important to consider the effect of the drug on both weight loss (or weight maintenance) and comorbidity, as well as any detrimental side-effects (14, 58).

Principles of drug treatment
In any discussion of the rational use of drugs for the treatment of obesity, it is important to understand the following:

- Currently approved drugs are best used in conjunction with diet and lifestyle management. Drugs used for weight management assist patient compliance with dietary, exercise and behaviour-change regimens.

- Weight-management drugs do not cure obesity; when they are discontinued, weight regain occurs.

- Drugs for weight management should be used under medical supervision.

- Drugs for weight management do not work if they are not taken (*59*). Weight regain can be expected when drugs are discontinued.

- Drug treatment should be considered part of a long-term management strategy for obesity tailored to the individual. Risks associated with drug treatment should be balanced against those of persistent obesity.

- Drug treatment should be continued only if it is considered to be safe and effective for a given patient. Current criteria in the United Kingdom suggest that the use of weight-management drugs for longer than 3 months should be considered only if a total weight loss of at least 10% has been achieved from the start of the episode of managed care (i.e. including weight loss achieved as a result of the obligatory 3–6 months of lifestyle intervention before drug treatment is initiated (*60*). However, this principle has been criticized as being unrealistic in most cases.

Drug treatment for obesity can be considered when patients:

— have a BMI >30 and treatment with diet, exercise and behaviour regimens has proved unsuccessful;
— have substantial comorbidities associated with a BMI >25 that have persisted in spite of an improved diet, exercise and behavioural treatment.

Weight-management drugs are not recommended for use in children as there are insufficient data on their effects on eating behaviour during the peripubertal period or in the longer term.

Types of drugs for weight management
Weight-management drugs can be broadly divided into two types — those that act on the central nervous system to influence feeding behaviour, appetite and other mechanisms, and peripherally acting drugs such as those that target the gastrointestinal system and inhibit absorption or enhance a feeling of fullness. As there is no published evidence to suggest that bulk-forming agents taken in a medicated form (e.g. methylcellulose) have any beneficial long-term effect in reducing weight, they are not discussed further here. However, increasing dietary fibre as part of dietary modification may have a role in energy restriction.

Weight-management drugs currently available in certain countries are summarized in Table 10.4. A number of them are considered in greater detail below. Many additional agents are currently under investigation.

In 1997 concerns were raised about the safety of two widely used weight-management drugs, fenfluramine and dexfenfluramine, be-

Table 10.4
Anti-obesity drugs currently available for use

Principal mode of action	Drug
Centrally acting:	
noradrenergic	Phentermine
combined serotonergic and noradrenergic	Sibutramine
Peripherally acting:	
lipase inhibitor	Tetrahydrolipostatin
Peripherally and centrally acting:	
thermogenic and anorectic	Ephedrine; caffeine

cause of their association with heart valve problems when used alone or in combination with phentermine. As a result of these concerns the manufacturer agreed to withdraw both treatments from the market. These drugs are therefore not considered in this report.

Efficacy of currently available drugs
A clinically useful drug for obesity treatment should have the following characteristics (*61*):

— demonstrated effectiveness in reducing body weight and weight-dependent disease;[1]
— tolerable and/or transient side-effects;
— no addictive properties;
— remains effective when used long-term;
— no major problems after many years of administration;
— known mechanisms of action(s);
— reasonable cost.

Ephedrine and caffeine combination. Data from a study by Astrup et al. (*62*) demonstrate the sustained effects of ephedrine in combination with caffeine on body weight when administered with a restrictive diet over a 1-year period. Although ephedrine and caffeine have thermogenic effects, around 75% of weight loss was attributed to the anorectic properties of this combination.

Tetrahydrolipstatin. Tetrahydrolipostatin is a pancreatic lipase inhibitor developed specifically for weight management. It blocks the cleavage of triglycerides in the gastrointestinal tract and thereby prevents

---

[1] Details of safe and efficacious dosages are beyond the scope of this report; appropriate medical references should be consulted. Drug approval agencies such as the Food and Drug Administration in the USA require drugs to produce at least 5% greater weight loss than a placebo, or to result in significantly more subjects achieving a 5–10% weight loss than can achieve a similar loss with a placebo.

the absorption of up to 30% of ingested dietary fat (*63*). Undigested fat is excreted unchanged in the faeces, causing an increase in intestinal side-effects (such as fatty/oily stools, abdominal pain and flatulence) especially if the ingested diet has a high fat content. Tetrahydrolipostatin has been shown to produce dose-dependent weight loss with improvements in total and LDL cholesterol and glucose tolerance in short-term trials (*64, 65*). It does not have the CNS side-effects of centrally acting drugs, but concern has been raised about the possibility of carotenoid malabsorption with extended use.

Phentermine. Phentermine acts as an anorexiant agent and original reports indicated good short-term weight loss when the drug was used in continuous or intermittent therapy for periods of up to 36 weeks (*66, 67*). However, side-effects such as insomnia, irritability, agitation, tension and anxiety occur in some patients and limit its use. There have been few recent trials of phentermine as a single anti-obesity agent and its widest use was in combination with fenfluramine before this agent was withdrawn from the market.[1]

Sibutramine. Sibutramine is a new drug developed for the treatment of obesity that combines the beneficial effects of serotonergic and adrenergic drugs. Controlled trials in obese patients have shown consistent results, and dose-related weight loss (at the optimum drug dose of 10–15 mg daily) was maintained for up to 12 months (*68, 69*). Weight loss is accompanied by a reduction in waist : hip ratio and by improvements in blood lipids and glycaemic control (*70*). Side-effects of sibutramine are moderate, and include nausea, dry mouth, constipation, dizziness and insomnia. Small increases in blood pressure and heart rate have also been reported in patients taking sibutramine, suggesting that these parameters need to be closely monitored. However, in longer trials, blood pressure has been shown to decrease with loss of weight in sibutramine-treated groups (*71*).

Drugs not appropriate for treatment of obesity per se
A number of drugs have a history of inappropriate and unsafe use for the promotion of weight loss (*58*). Diuretics, human chorionic gonadotropin (HCG), amfetamine, dexamfetamine and thyroxine are not treatments for obesity and should not be used to achieve weight loss. Thyroxine should never be prescribed for obesity, only

---

[1] Concerns about the possible side-effects (heart valve problems) associated with the use of fenfluramine and dexfenfluramine, either alone or in combination with phentermine, led to the withdrawal of these drugs from the market.

for biochemically proven hypothyroidism. Metformin and acarbose may be useful in the management of obese NIDDM patients but have no proven efficacy for obesity alone.

Fluoxetine, serraline and other selective serotonin reuptake inhibitors have a legitimate use in the treatment of a depressive condition associated with obesity but not for obesity itself. They may help some patients lose weight and are preferred to tricyclic agents for overweight depressed patients. Fluoxetine is licensed in certain countries for the management of bulimia nervosa.

Appropriateness of long-term drug treatment
While the clinical tolerance of most drugs appears to be acceptable, their long-term use raises some safety concerns. The importance of this issue has been highlighted by the recent reports of heart valve problems in a small number of patients taking fenfluramine and dexfenfluramine (72).

As with drugs prescribed for long-term treatment in other chronic diseases (e.g. hypertension, NIDDM), the risk associated with long-term drug use for weight management must be weighed against the potential benefits for each individual. In addition, weight-management drugs should be withdrawn in poor responders after 1–3 months of evaluation. Preliminary research suggests that it is possible to identify patients at an early stage of treatment who are most likely to respond (71). However, more research is needed before criteria can be recommended. Long-term outcomes also need to be assessed.

Comparative trials are necessary as new drugs are introduced for therapy, particularly with regard to reduction in comorbidities.

10.5.5 Gastric surgery
Surgery is now considered to be the most effective way of reducing weight, and maintaining weight loss, in severely obese (BMI >35) and very severely obese (BMI >40) subjects. On the basis of cost/kg of weight lost, surgical treatment has been estimated, after 4 years, to be less expensive than any other treatment (estimates cited in reference 73).

Surgical procedures
A variety of different surgical methods are available for the treatment of obesity, generally based on restriction of energy intake, on malabsorption or maldigestion of food, or on a combination of both. It is now agreed that vertical-banded gastroplasty and Roux-en-Y gastric bypass are effective and safe, with follow-up of 15 years or more in some series. The full evaluation of long-term safety and efficacy of biliopancreatic bypass and laparoscopic adaptations of restrictive

(e.g. adjustable banding) and combined procedures is still awaited. Intestinal bypass surgery is no longer recommended as a primary surgical method of treating obesity (16, 74).

Patient selection

Patients should be selected for surgery in accordance with the following principles:

- Non-surgical treatment including dietary measures and weight-reducing drugs should be tried first.

- Gastrointestinal surgery for obesity should be used only on well informed and motivated patients with acceptable operative risks.

- Patients should have a BMI >40, or >35 together with high-risk, life-threatening comorbid conditions.

- Surgery should be undertaken only by an experienced surgeon in an appropriate clinical setting under expert medical surveillance, and with access to ventilator facilities and the support of a multidisciplinary team.

Improvements after surgery

Weight loss of more than 20 kg generally occurs within 12 months of operations, although some weight is regained within 5–15 years. Analysis of the results of the SOS study in Sweden showed weight losses of 30–40 kg over 2 years depending on the surgical procedure used (75).

Gastric bypass surgery ameliorates obesity-related morbidity in the majority of obese patients. In the SOS study, surgical treatment produced remission of NIDDM in 68% of obese patients and of hypertension in 43%. For those who did not have risk factors at baseline, a 30-kg weight loss was associated with a 14-fold risk reduction for NIDDM, and 3–4-fold risk reductions with respect to the development of hypertension and other cardiovascular risk factors (75). In addition, surgical treatment has been shown to prevent progression of impaired glucose tolerance to NIDDM (76) and to reduce mortality from diabetes 4–5-fold.

Quality of life measures, including employability, median wage, number of sick days, social interaction, mobility, self-image, assertiveness and depression, are also improved in the majority of patients after antiobesity surgery. Recently, patients in the surgical intervention group of the SOS study reported marked improvements in social interaction, perceived health, mood, anxiety, depression and obesity-specific problems compared with controls (75).

Risks associated with surgery

Risks associated with gastric surgery include micronutrient deficiencies, neuropathy, postoperative complications, "dumping syndrome" and late postoperative depression (*74*). It has been suggested, however, that most of the complications associated with this type of surgery, unlike most other surgery, are treatable with behavioural therapy. Kral (*77*), for example, notes that the vomiting seen in approximately 10% of patients after surgery is due more to eating behaviour than to stenosis or stricture of the gastroplasty stoma.

Operative mortality in experienced centres is a fraction of the mortality observed in unoperated patients and in those remaining on waiting lists for operations.[1]

Liposuction of unwanted subcutaneous fat depots is being used extensively for cosmetic reasons but offers no medical benefit in terms of comorbidities linked to obesity.

10.5.6 *Traditional medicine*

Many countries have traditional medical systems that provide treatment in addition to, or in place of, conventional medical services. Traditional treatments for a range of illnesses, including obesity, are often available and are commonly used by people in developing countries. Although there are limited data on the efficacy of the medicines used, there is anecdotal evidence of their potential value. For example, some preparations of plant products containing capsaicin have been shown to increase energy expenditure by increasing thermogenesis (*78*). More research is required to evaluate the potential use of such traditional remedies.

Caution is necessary, however. A variety of herbal preparations widely promoted by commercial organizations as traditional remedies have been shown to be of little medical value and, in some cases, to contain dangerous substances.

10.5.7 *Other treatments*

A number of other treatments have been promoted as effective in the management of weight but very little objective research has been done on them. In uncontrolled trials, acupuncture and yoga have been shown to assist weight loss, and an assessment by Rand & Stunkard indicates that support from psychoanalysts can produce weight loss

---

[1] Kral JG. Surgery. In: Guy-Grand B, ed. *Management of obesity and overweight*, 1996. Background paper prepared by Obesity Management subgroup of International Obesity Task Force.

and maintenance in their patients (79). There is no evidence that hypnotherapy for obesity is any more effective in the long term than the usual diet and behavioural treatment programmes (80). However, hypnosis may improve self-image and possibly help patients to adhere to a prescribed diet (81).

10.6 Management of obesity in childhood and adolescence

The objectives of weight-management strategies for children differ from those for adults because consideration needs to be given to the physical and intellectual development of the child. Whereas adult treatment may target weight loss, child treatment targets the prevention of weight gain. Lean body mass increases as children age, so that reducing fat mass or keeping it constant will result in a normalization of body weight.

The treatment of obese children to prevent them from becoming obese adults can be classified as targeted prevention (see section 8), because childhood obesity substantially increases the risk of adult obesity (see section 7). Treatment of childhood obesity should therefore be considered together with selective preventive strategies aimed at high-risk groups of children as well as part of a universal approach to the community-wide prevention of childhood obesity.

10.6.1 Evidence that treatment of childhood obesity prevents later adult obesity

Evidence that the treatment of obesity in children can be successfully managed over the period from childhood through adolescence to adulthood is provided by the work of Epstein and colleagues. In a series of four studies, data from 158 families with children at high risk for significant adult obesity were followed up 10 years after their initial treatment. At the time of the initial treatment, the children were between 6 and 12 years of age, averaged 40–50% overweight and, with the exception of one study group, had at least one obese parent. Different treatment conditions were investigated but all involved a diet plan together with intensive group behaviour modification over an 8–12 week period, followed by monthly maintenance sessions for 6–12 months (55).

After 10 years of follow-up, six out of nine actively treated groups showed a net reduction in percentage overweight of between 10% and 20% (Fig. 10.3). Inclusion of a parent with the child in treatment and introduction of exercise into the basic diet and behaviour change programme enhanced the long-term effects.

It may be premature to make broad generalizations about the efficacy of obesity treatment in children, especially as it may not always be

Figure 10.3

Changes in percentage overweight after 5 and 10 years of follow-up for obese children randomly assigned to 10 interventions across four studies[a]

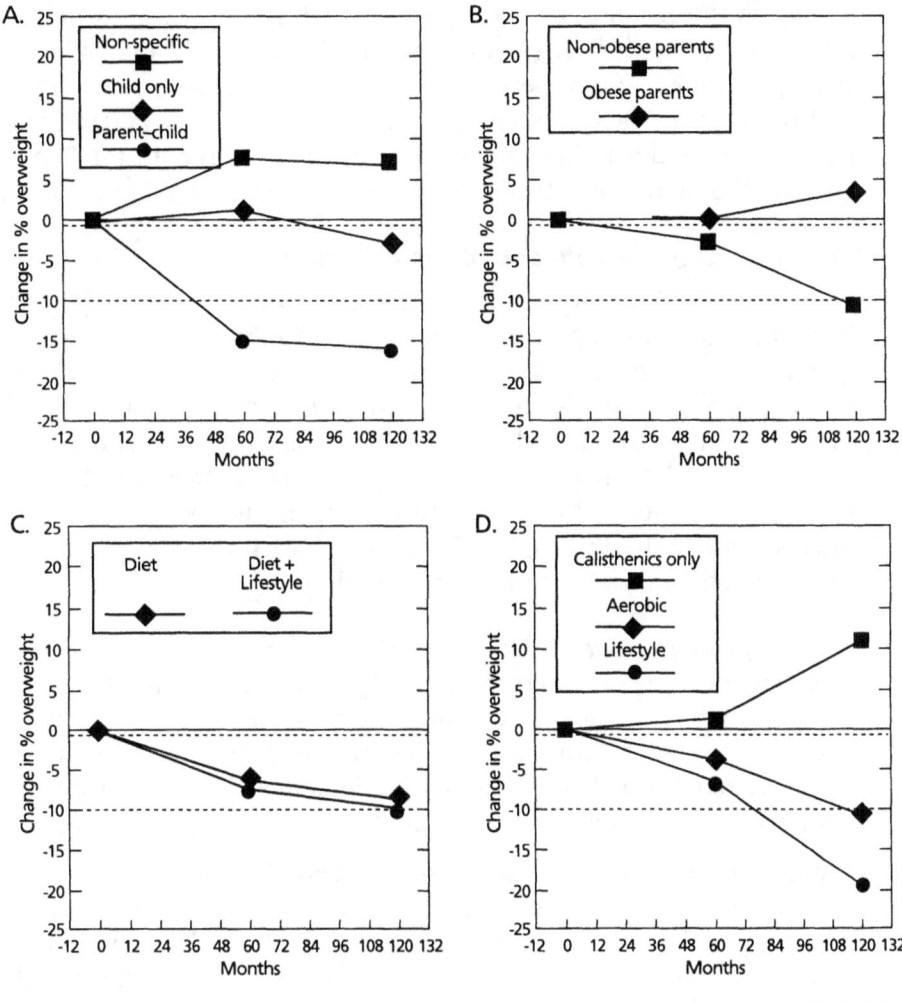

WHO 98278

The 95% confidence interval for the total sample of children is represented by dotted lines. The interventions all contained a diet and behavioural change component plus the specific approaches under investigation. In the four separate studies in which Epstein et al. examined the impact of different interventions for obesity management in overweight children, all had the same basic diet and behavioural change intervention for 8–12 weeks and monthly review for 6–12 months. Study A compared results for children alone, children with one parent, and nonspecific directions. Study B compared relative weight changes in children of obese and non-obese parents. Study C examined the benefit of adding lifestyle (unstructured exercise) to a diet programme. Study D compared the effectiveness of different forms of exercise in aiding weight control. Both children and parents were followed up 5 and 10 years after the initial programme. The results show excellent long-term benefits and demonstrate the value of family support and a positive family environment and the value of unstructured exercise in weight control in children.

[a] Adapted from reference *55* with the permission of the publisher and authors. Copyright 1994 by the American Psychological Association.

feasible to provide the high level of support given in the studies mentioned above, and the children in these studies were recruited from largely white, middle-class, two-parent families. However, they provide grounds for optimism in that comprehensive behavioural treatments appear to offer enduring benefits to obese children. A longitudinal trial to determine whether results like those achieved by Epstein and colleagues can be replicated at other sites and in other populations, and whether tangible health benefits, in both the health and social domains, can be demonstrated, would be highly desirable.

10.6.2 *Treatment of overweight and obese children*

Overweight and obesity during childhood are among the major risk factors for the development of obesity in adulthood, since approximately 30% of obese children become obese adults (*82*). Childhood obesity affects health, resulting in reduced fitness, increased blood pressure and adverse blood lipid levels (see section 4). In addition to the immediate health effects, obesity in adolescence increases the risk of adult morbidity and mortality 50 years later, independently of the effects of adult obesity (*83, 84*). These are powerful reasons for developing effective obesity therapies for children.

Reducing energy intake and improving dietary quality
It is generally recommended that only small reductions in energy intake should be made in the diet of the overweight child, as an adequate intake of both energy and nutrients is required by children to ensure that normal growth and development are not compromised. Treatment is recommended only for children over 6 years of age.

Limiting portion sizes of energy-dense foods is a useful method of reducing energy intake in obese children. This can be achieved by preparing and serving smaller quantities of such foods or by encouraging free consumption of fruits and vegetables so that energy density is reduced without imposing dietary restrictions. However, only limited data support the suggestion that an increased variety of food intake results in a decreased intake of energy-dense foods (*85*).

Limiting take-away and ready-prepared foods, which tend to be particularly high in fat and energy-dense, may also help to control energy intake. These foods are making increasingly large contributions to the energy intake of children and adolescents around the world (*86–88*). Children should also be encouraged to eat fewer high-fat snacks, and to avoid obtaining a large proportion of total energy from sweetened beverages or even to choose unsweetened drinks or water. One study on prepubertal children in which an attempt was made to reduce fat intake over 12 months did not achieve weight loss or reductions in weight gain in the target group despite achieving some dietary change (*89*). However, the children concerned were not obese.

Promoting the consumption of food high in complex carbohydrates, low in fat and low in energy density is likely to be important in preventing excessive energy consumption in children. It is important to encourage all children, whether overweight or not, to adopt healthy eating habits from an early age and to continue them into adulthood.

Increasing physical activity

Research on the value of exercise in treating childhood obesity is very limited, and much remains to be elucidated, particularly in relation to the long-term benefits of physical activity in the control of weight through childhood and adolescence. Available evidence suggests that exercise alone is not sufficient for the effective management of childhood obesity, and that a combination of diet and exercise is more effective for long-term control (*90*).

All children should be encouraged to be as active as possible. However, it appears that energy expenditure can be increased more effectively through increased general activity and play rather than through competitive sport and structured exercise (*90*). Obese children are particularly sensitive to peer attitudes towards body shape and exercise performance, and have the same problems as adults in adhering to long-term exercise programmes. Since this tends to limit their willingness to be involved in team sports (*91*), it is likely to be counterproductive to pay too much attention to the reintroduction of competitive sports at schools to improve the poor levels of physical activity in schoolchildren.

Some of the methods that have been used to improve adherence to exercise programmes in adults may be equally useful for children. These include making the activity enjoyable by increasing the choice of type and level of activities, as well as by providing positive reinforcement of their achievements during exercise rather than only after the successful completion of the exercise session (*90*).

Increasing physical activity in children is associated with benefits other than raising energy expenditure. For example, being active may compete with snacking and thereby make adherence to a diet easier. In addition, resistance training may have effects on body composition that complement, or are superior to, those of aerobic exercise alone; resistance training will lead to an increase in lean body mass, thus increasing metabolic rate and total daily energy expenditure, and may have positive effects on body image (*90*). Thus, although improvement in aerobic fitness is likely to be beneficial, it should not be an overriding concern.

Reducing time spent in sedentary behaviour
New research is beginning to indicate that the amount of time spent in sedentary behaviour or inactivity may play an even more important role than low levels of physical activity in the genesis of children's weight problems. The rapid rise in overweight in childhood has been accompanied by an explosion of non-active leisure pursuits for children such as computer and video games. Television is the principal cause of inactivity for most children and adolescents in developed countries and has been linked to the prevalence of obesity (*92, 93*). Television viewing is also associated with increased intake of high-energy snacks (*93, 94*). It is of particular interest that the study by Epstein et al. (*95*) clearly showed that short-term weight losses were greater in a group of children who were instructed to reduce sedentary behaviour than in children who were encouraged to increase exercise. Reducing physical inactivity also resulted in improved maintenance of weight loss and a more positive attitude towards vigorous activity.

Role of drugs and surgery
Limited information is available on the use of aggressive forms of treatment such as drugs and surgery for children and adolescents, although such treatment may be indicated in children with potentially fatal complications of obesity.

10.6.3 *Obesity-management programmes for children*

Three main types of obesity-management programmes aimed at children can be identified — family-based, school-based, and primary-care-based programmes. These are considered in detail in the following paragraphs.

Family-based programmes
As the family environment is one of the strongest influences on a child's risk of obesity, a logical setting for childhood obesity prevention and management would appear to be the families of susceptible children. Indeed, the provision of appropriate education on eating and lifestyles to parents has been shown to significantly reduce the prevalence of obesity in children of participating families for periods of 3 months to 3 years when compared with families not receiving advice and support (*96*). Parental attitudes, purchase and presentation of food, modelling of eating and exercise habits, and support

for active leisure pursuits can all affect a child's eating and exercise pattern.

Strong evidence for the important role of family support in childhood obesity and weight-management programmes comes from a number of successful interventions. Flodmark et al. found improved weight loss or weight maintenance in children aged 10–11 years treated with family therapy when compared with those treated alone (97), and Wadden et al. obtained similar results in African-American teen-age girls (98). A more detailed analysis by Epstein et al. (55) suggested that weight regulation is improved if at least one parent is treated together with the child. When the effect of targeting an over-weight child alone was compared with that of targeting a child and a parent together, the latter showed significantly less weight gain at 5 years follow-up, and were still below the relative weight (weight corrected for height) at which they started the study at 10 years follow-up (Fig. 10.3B). Furthermore, children of non-obese parents were better able to obtain and maintain reductions in relative weight (Fig. 10.3C). Epstein's findings are especially important because relative weight was maintained throughout adolescence when weight gain can be a major problem. Other investigators have also found improved effectiveness of family-based programmes in preventing the progression of childhood obesity.

By targeting obesity-prevention measures on the family of susceptible children there is the added advantage that all members of the family are likely to benefit. This helps to increase social support and to reduce the feelings of isolation that may develop when one child is treated separately from the rest of the family. In addition, parents are able to exert a higher degree of external control over the child's eating and activity patterns under these circumstances (54).

School-based programmes
The introduction of obesity-prevention programmes in schools is justified for a number of reasons. A large proportion of children attend school (although this percentage varies from country to country) and much of a child's eating and exercise takes place in this setting. Schools can also assist in identifying children who may be at risk of obesity through educational programmes and visits to the school doctor at key developmental stages. Furthermore, the start of schooling corresponds to a period of increased risk for excessive weight gain as children begin to become independent and vary their diet and activity patterns in line with their new circumstances.

The results of various school-based obesity-intervention programmes targeting high-risk children and adolescents suggest that these can be successfully implemented and can reach substantial numbers of children in need of obesity prevention (*99–101*). Obese children in treatment groups have consistently shown greater reductions in percentage overweight than untreated obese controls. Results over periods of 3–6 months are modestly encouraging and would seem to justify additional research in this area.

Increasing physical activity through integrating regular exercise programmes into school curricula is a strategy that has often been suggested as an effective means of improving the weight and health status of children (*102, 103*). The evaluation of a 2-year project in South Australia, where a 50-minute session of daily physical activity was introduced into a number of primary schools, demonstrated that children who took part in the programme were fitter, slimmer and had lower diastolic blood pressure (boys only) than their non-participating counterparts (*104*). A subsequent study in which classroom lessons on nutrition and physical health were included was also able to demonstrate improvements in indices of fitness and body fat levels (*105*). Similar programmes have been introduced in schools in the USA (*90*) and Singapore (*106*), where short-term results appear promising. However, despite these beneficial results, the maintenance of these programmes within the school curricula in the long term has proved difficult due to competition for school time, the need for teacher/adult supervision, and financial limitations.

Primary-care-based programmes
The delivery of childhood obesity-management programmes through primary care has received little formal assessment so far, and its potential role appears to be undervalued and underutilized (*16*). One general practice in the United Kingdom has had some success in reducing obesity by providing healthy eating advice to pregnant women and their children. Obesity prevalence was only 2% within the patient sample compared with 8% among patients who did not receive advice (*5*).

Frequent contact with health professionals from an early age has been identified as one of the most important strategies for the effective management of overweight and obese children, which suggests that similar strategies might be equally effective in prevention (*107*). Regular assessment and contact through home visits provide an excellent opportunity for education about the potential lifestyle risk factors associated with obesity, as well as for advice, encouragement and support to help parents to adopt healthy household eating and exercise patterns at an early stage in life. It has been suggested that obesity prevention should start with appropriate advice about breast feeding, weaning and diet for toddlers (*108*). In many countries, child health nurses already play a crucial role in monitoring the development of infants and young children.

Special considerations in the management of childhood obesity
The value of prudent attempts to prevent excessive weight gain in normal-weight children, or to reduce weight gain in children who are already obese, is evident. Consideration of the following issues is of vital importance when developing interventions aimed at preventing or treating obesity in young children.

- *Risk of malnutrition.* As adequate nutrition is essential for promoting healthy growth, only small reductions in overall energy intake are recommended where such an approach is advised.

- *Risk of eating disorders.* It is important that interventions do not encourage the type of dietary restraint that has been linked to the development of eating disorders and other psychological problems (*54*).

- *Risk of isolation.* It is important that overweight children are not ostracized and made to feel any more different from their peers than is necessary, either at home or at school (*84*). The message that everyone is potentially at risk of obesity may help, but there is also a need to generate family awareness of the need for healthier lifestyles without suggesting that the one and only goal is to lose weight.

References

1. **Forster JL et al.** Preventing weight gain in adults: a pound of prevention. *Health Psychology*, 1988, 7:515–525.

2. **Jeffery RW, French SA.** Preventing weight gain in adults: design, methods and one year results from the Pound of Prevention study. *International Journal of Obesity and Related Metabolic Disorders*, 1997, 21:457–464.

3. World Health Organization European Collaborative Group. European collaborative trial of multifactorial prevention of coronary heart disease: final report on the 6-year results. *Lancet*, 1986, i:869–872.

4. **Jeffery RW et al.** Strengthening behavioral interventions for weight loss: a randomized trial of food provision and monetary incentives. *Journal of Consulting and Clinical Psychology*, 1993, 61:1038–1045.

5. **Craddock D.** *Obesity and its management*, 3rd ed. Edinburgh, Churchill Livingstone, 1978:160–173.

6. OXCHECK Study Group, Imperial Cancer Research Fund. Effectiveness of health checks conducted by nurses in primary care: final results of the OXCHECK Study. *British Medical Journal*, 1995, 310:1099–1104.

7. **Wood DA et al.** A randomised controlled trial evaluating cardiovascular screening and intervention in general practice: principal results of the British Family Heart Study. *British Medical Journal*, 1994, **308**:313–320.

8. **Rössner S.** Factors determining the long-term outcome of obesity treatment. In: Björntorp P, Brodoff BN, eds. *Obesity.* Philadelphia, Lippincott, 1992:712–719.

9. **Goldstein DJ.** Beneficial health effects of modest weight loss. *International Journal of Obesity and Related Metabolic Disorders*, 1992, **16**:397–415.

10. **Williamson DF et al.** Prospective study of intentional weight loss and mortality in never-smoking overweight US white women aged 40–64 years. *American Journal of Epidemiology*, 1995, **141**:1128–1141.

11. **Wing RR et al.** Food provision vs structured meal plans in the behavioural treatment of obesity. *International Journal of Obesity and Related Metabolic Disorders*, 1996, **20**:56–62.

12. **Sonne-Holm S et al.** Independent effects of weight change and attained body weight on prevalence of arterial hypertension in obese and non-obese men. *British Medical Journal* 1989, **299**:767–770.

13. **Wilson GT.** Relation of dieting and voluntary weight loss to psychological functioning and binge eating. *Annals of Internal Medicine*, 1993, **119**:727–730.

14. National Taskforce on the Prevention and Treatment of Obesity. Long-term pharmacotherapy in the management of obesity. *Journal of the American Medical Association*, 1996, **276**:1907–1915.

15. Committee to develop criteria for evaluating the outcomes of approaches to prevent and treat obesity within the Food and Nutrition Board of the Institute of Medicine. In: Thomas PR, ed. *Weighing the options: criteria for evaluating weight-management programs.* Washington, DC, National Academy Press, 1995, 234–235.

16. *Obesity in Scotland. Integrating prevention with weight management. A national clinical guideline recommended for use in Scotland.* Edinburgh, Scottish Intercollegiate Guidelines Network, 1996.

17. *Shape Up America: guidance for treatment of adult obesity.* Bethesda, MD, American Obesity Association (AOA), 1997.

18. **Ferro-Luzzi A, Martino L.** Obesity and physical activity. In: Chadwick DJ, Cardew GC, eds. *The origins and consequences of obesity.* Chichester, Wiley, 1996:207–227 (Ciba Foundation Symposium 201).

19. **Buzzard IM, Sievert YA.** Research priorities and recommendations for dietary assessment methodology. First International Conference on Dietary Assessment Methods. *American Journal of Clinical Nutrition*, 1994, **59**(1 Suppl.):275S–280S.

20. **St Jeor ST.** Measurement of food intake. In: Brownell KD, Fairburn CG, eds. *Eating disorders and obesity: a comprehensive handbook.* New York, Guilford Press, 1995, 100–104.

21. **Rössner S.** Cessation of cigarette smoking and body weight increase. *Acta Medica Scandinavica*, 1986, 219:1–2.

22. Fitzgibbon ML, Kirschenbaum DS. Heterogeneity of clinical presentation among obese individuals seeking treatment. *Addictive Behaviors*, 1990, 15:291–295.

23. Wadden TA, Foster GD. Behavioural assessment and treatment of markedly obese patients. In: Wadden TA, Van Itallie TB, eds. *Treatment of the seriously obese patient*. New York, Guilford Press, 1992:290–330.

24. Meisler JG, St Jeor S. Summary and recommendations from the American Health Foundation's Expert Panel on Healthy Weight. *American Journal of Clinical Nutrition*, 1996, 63(3 Suppl.):474S–477S.

25. Jeffery RW et al. Monetary contracts in weight control: effectiveness of group and individual contracts of varying size. *Journal of Consulting and Clinical Psychology*, 1983, 51:242–248.

26. Cousins JH et al. Family versus individually orientated intervention for weight loss in Mexican American women. *Public Health Reports*, 1992, 107:549–555.

27. Perri MG, Nezu AM, Viegner BJ. *Improving the long-term management of obesity*. New York, Wiley Bioscience, 1992.

28. Brownell KD, Wadden TA. The heterogeneity of obesity: fitting treatments to individuals. *Behaviour Research and Therapy*, 1991, 22:153–177.

29. Black DR, Threlfall WE. Partner weight status and subject weight loss: implications for cost-effective programs and public health. *Addictive Behaviors*, 1989, 14:279–289.

30. Pratt CA. Development of a screening questionnaire to study attrition in weight-control programs. *Psychological Reports*, 1989, 64:1007–1016.

31. Epstein LH et al. Ten-year follow-up of behavioral, family-based treatment for obese children. *Journal of the American Medical Association*, 1990, 264:2519–2523.

32. Stunkard AJ. An overview of current treatments for obesity. In: Wadden TA, Van Itallie TB, eds. *Treatment of the seriously obese patient*. New York, Guilford Press, 1992.

33. Bennett W. Dietary treatments of obesity. *Annals of the New York Academy of Sciences*, 1987, 499:250–263.

34. Frost G et al. A new method of energy prescription to improve weight loss. *Journal of Human Nutrition and Dietetics*, 1991, 4:369–373.

35. Lean ME, James WPT. Prescription of diabetic diets in the 1980s. *Lancet*, 1986, i:723–725.

36. Prentice AM et al. Metabolism or appetite? Questions of energy balance with particular reference to obesity. *Journal of Human Nutrition and Dietetics*, 1989, 2:95–104.

37. Lean ME et al. Weight loss with high and low carbohydrate 1200 kcal diets in free living women. *European Journal of Clinical Nutrition*, 1997, 51(4):243–248.

38. Astrup A et al. The role of low fat diets and fat substitutes in body weight management. What have we learned from clinical studies? *Journal of the American Dietetic Association*, 1997, 97(7 Suppl.):S82–S87.

39. **Toubro S, Astrup A.** Randomised comparisons of diets for maintaining obese subjects' weight after major weight loss: ad lib, low fat, high carbohydrate diet v fixed energy intake. *British Medical Journal*, 1997, 314:29–34.

40. **Blackburn GL.** Comparison of medically supervised and unsupervised approaches to weight loss and control. *Annals of Internal Medicine*, 1993, 119:714–718.

41. **Wadden TA.** Treatment of obesity by moderate and severe caloric restriction. Results of clinical research trials. *Annals of Internal Medicine*, 1993, **119**:688–693.

42. **Wadden TA, Foster GD, Letizia KA.** One-year behavioral treatment of obesity: comparison of moderate and severe caloric restriction and the effects of maintenance therapy. *Journal of Consulting and Clinical Psychology*, 1994, **62**:165–171.

43. **James WPT.** Dietary aspects of obesity. *Postgraduate Medical Journal*, 1984, **60**(Suppl. 3):50–55.

44. **Wadden TA et al.** Treatment of obesity by very low calorie diet, behavior therapy, and their combination: a five-year perspective. *International Journal of Obesity*, 1989, **13**(Suppl. 2):39–46.

45. **Skender ML et al.** Comparison of 2-year weight loss trends in behavioral treatments of obesity: diet, exercise, and combination interventions. *Journal of the American Dietetic Association*, 1996, **96**:342–346.

46. **Garrow JS, Summerbell CD.** Meta-analysis: effect of exercise, with or without dieting, on the body composition of overweight subjects. *European Journal of Clinical Nutrition*, 1995, **49**:1–10.

47. **Wing RR.** Behavioral treatment of severe obesity. *American Journal of Clinical Nutrition*, 1992, **55**(2 Suppl.):545S–555S.

48. *Physical activity and health: a report of the Surgeon General.* Washington, DC, US Department of Health and Human Services, 1996.

49. *Health Update 5. Physical activity.* London, Health Education Authority, 1995.

50. **Saris WHM.** Physical activity and body weight regulation. In: Bouchard C, Bray GA, eds. *Regulation of body weight. Biological and behavioural mechanisms.* Chichester, Wiley, 1996:135–148.

51. **Després JP, Lamarche B.** Low-intensity endurance exercise training, plasma lipoproteins and the risk of coronary heart disease. *Journal of Internal Medicine*, 1994, **236**:7–22.

52. **James WPT, Schofield EC.** *Human energy requirements. A manual for planners and nutritionists.* Oxford, Oxford University Press, 1990.

53. **Hillsdon M et al.** Randomised controlled trials of physical activity promotion in free living populations: a review. *Journal of Epidemiology and Community Health*, 1995, **49**:448–453.

54. **Wilson GT.** Behavioral treatment of childhood obesity: theoretical and practical implications. *Health Psychology*, 1994, **13**:371–372.

55. **Epstein LH et al.** Ten-year outcomes of behavioral family-based treatment for childhood obesity. *Health Psychology*, 1994, **13**:373–383.

56. **Wilson GT.** Behavioral approaches to the treatment of obesity. In: Brownell KD, Fairburn CG, eds. *Eating disorders and obesity; a comprehensive handbook*. New York, Guilford Press, 1995:479–483.

57. **Guy-Grand B.** A new approach to the treatment of obesity. A discussion. *Annals of the New York Academy of Sciences*, 1987, **499**:313–317.

58. Working Party on Obesity Management. *Overweight and obese patients: principles of management with particular reference to the use of drugs.* London, Royal College of Physicians, 1997.

59. **Bray GA.** Use and abuse of appetite-suppressant drugs in the treatment of obesity. *Annals of Internal Medicine*, 1993, **119**:707–713.

60. *Clinical management of overweight and obese patients with particular reference to the use of drugs.* London, Royal College of Physicians, 1998.

61. **Guy-Grand B.** Long term pharmacotherapy in the management of obesity. In: Björntorp P, Rössner S, eds. *From theory to practice: obesity in Europe: 88.* London, John Libbey, 1989:311–318.

62. **Astrup A et al.** The effect and safety of an ephedrine/caffeine compound compared to ephedrine, caffeine and placebo in obese subjects on an energy restricted diet. A double blind trial. *International Journal of Obesity and Related Metabolic Disorders*, 1992, **16**:269–277.

63. **Hauptman JB, Jeunet FS, Hartmann D.** Initial studies in humans with the novel gastrointestinal lipase inhibitor Ro 18-0647 (tetrahydrolipstatin). *American Journal of Clinical Nutrition*, 1992, **55**(1 Suppl.):309S–313S.

64. **Drent ML, van der Veen EA.** Lipase inhibition: a novel concept in the treatment of obesity. *International Journal of Obesity and Related Metabolic Disorders*, 1993, **17**:241–244.

65. **Drent ML et al.** Orlistat (Ro 18-0647), a lipase inhibitor, in the treatment of human obesity: a multiple dose study. *International Journal of Obesity and Related Metabolic Disorders*, 1995, **19**:221–226.

66. **Munro JF et al.** Comparison of continuous and intermittent anorectic therapy in obesity. *British Medical Journal*, 1968, **1**:352–354.

67. **Steel JM, Munro JF, Duncan LJP.** A comparative trial of different regimens of fenfluramine and phentermine in obesity. *The Practitioner*, 1973, **211**:232–236.

68. **Bray GA et al.** Sibutramine — dose response and long-term efficacy in weight loss, a double-blind study. *International Journal of Obesity and Related Metabolic Disorders*, 1994, **18**(Suppl. 2):60.

69. **Jones SP et al.** Long term weight loss with sibutramine. *International Journal of Obesity and Related Metabolic Disorders*, 1995, **19**(Suppl. 2):41.

70. **Griffiths J et al.** Sibutramine in the treatment of overweight non-insulin-dependent diabetics. *International Journal of Obesity and Related Metabolic Disorders*, 1995, **19**(Suppl. 2):41.

71. **Lean ME.** Sibutramine — a review of clinical efficacy. *International Journal of Obesity and Related Metabolic Disorders*, 1997, **21**(Suppl. 1):S30–S36.

72. Cannistra LB, Davis SM, Bauman AG. Valvular heart disease associated with dexfenfluramine. *New England Journal of Medicine*, 1997, **337**:636.

73. Kral J. Surgical treatment of obesity. In Wadden TA, Van Itallie TB, eds. *Treatment of the seriously obese patient*. New York, Guilford Press, 1995:496–506.

74. Gastrointestinal surgery for severe obesity. Proceedings of a National Institutes of Health Consensus Development Conference. *American Journal of Clinical Nutrition*, 1992, **55**(2 Suppl.):S487–S619.

75. Sjöström L, Marbro K, Sjöström D. Costs and benefits when treating obesity. *International Journal of Obesity and Related Metabolic Disorders*, 1995, **19**(Suppl. 6):S9–S12.

76. Long SD et al. Weight loss in severely obese subjects prevents the progression of impaired glucose tolerance to type-II diabetes. A longitudinal interventional study. *Diabetes Care*, 1994, **17**:372–375.

77. Kral JG. Side-effects, complications and problems in anti-obesity surgery. *International Journal of Obesity and Related Metabolic Disorders*, 1994, **18**(Suppl. 2):86.

78. Yoshioka M et al. Effects of red-pepper diet on the energy metabolism in men. *Journal of Nutritional Science and Vitaminology*, 1995, **41**:647–656.

79. Rand CS, Stunkard AJ. Obesity and psychoanalysis: treatment and four-year follow-up. *American Journal of Psychiatry*, 1983, **140**:1140–1144.

80. Mott T Jr, Roberts J. Obesity and hypnosis: a review of the literature. *American Journal of Clinical Hypnosis*, 1979, **22**:3–7.

81. Collins JK. Hypnosis: body image and weight control. In: Touyz S, Beaumont P, eds. *Eating disorders: prevalence and treatment*. Baltimore, MD, Williams & Wilkins, 1985:105–116.

82. Dietz WH. Therapeutic strategies in childhood obesity. *Hormone Research*, 1993, **39**(Suppl. 3):86–90.

83. Dietz WH. Childhood obesity. In: Björntorp P, Brodoff BN, eds. *Obesity*. Philadelphia, Lippincott, 1992, 606–609.

84. Must A et al. Long-term morbidity and mortality of overweight adolescents. A follow-up of the Harvard Growth Study of 1922 to 1935. *New England Journal of Medicine*, 1992, **327**:1350–1355.

85. Keendy E, Goldberg J. What are American children eating? Implications for public policy. *Nutrition Reviews*, 1995, **53**:111–126.

86. McKenzie J. Social changes and the food industry. *Nutrition Reviews*, 1982, **40**(Suppl.):13–17.

87. Department of Health. *The diets of British schoolchildren*. London, Her Majesty's Stationery Office, 1989 (Reports of Health and Social Subjects, No. 39).

88. Crawley HF. The energy, nutrient and food intakes of teenagers aged 16–17 years in Britain. 1. Energy, macronutrients and non-starch polysaccharides. *British Journal of Nutrition*, 1993, **70**:15–26.

89. Efficacy and safety of lowering dietary intake of fat and cholesterol in children with elevated low-density lipoprotein cholesterol. The Dietary

Intervention Study in Children (DISC). *Journal of the American Medical Association*, 1995, **273**:1429–1435.

90. **Epstein LH.** Exercise in the treatment of childhood obesity. *International Journal of Obesity and Related Metabolic Disorders*, 1995, **19**(Suppl. 4):S117–S121.

91. **Court JM.** Strategies for the management of obesity in children and adolescents. In: Hills AP, Wahlqvist ML, eds. *Exercise and obesity*. London, Smith Gordon, 1994:181–195.

92. **Dietz WH Jr, Gortmaker SL.** Do we fatten our children at the television set? Obesity and television viewing in children and adolescents. *Pediatrics*, 1985, **75**:807–812.

93. **Gortmaker SL et al.** Television viewing as a cause of increasing adiposity among children in the United States, 1986–1990. *Archives of Pediatrics and Adolescent Medicine*, 1996, **150**:356–362.

94. **Dietz WH Jr.** Prevention of childhood obesity. *Pediatric Clinics of North America*, 1986, **33**:823–833.

95. **Epstein LH et al.** Effects of decreasing sedentary behaviour and increasing activity on weight changes in obese children. *Health Psychology*, 1995, **14**:109–115.

96. **Pisacano JC et al.** An attempt at prevention of obesity in infancy. *Pediatrics*, 1978, **61**:360–364.

97. **Flodmark CE et al.** Prevention of progress to severe obesity in a group of obese schoolchildren treated with family therapy. *Pediatrics*, 1993, **91**:880–884.

98. **Wadden TA et al.** Obesity in black adolescent girls: a controlled clinical trial of treatment by diet, behavior modification, and parental support. *Pediatrics*, 1990, **85**:345–352.

99. **Seltzer CC, Mayer J.** An effective weight control program in a public school system. *American Journal of Public Health and the Nations' Health*, 1970, **60**:679–689.

100. **Foster GD, Wadden TA, Brownell KD.** Peer-led program for the treatment and prevention of obesity in the schools. *Journal of Consulting and Clinical Psychiatry*, 1985, **53**:538–540.

101. **Resnicow K.** School-based obesity prevention. Population versus high-risk interventions. *Annals of the New York Academy of Sciences*, 1993, **699**:154–166.

102. **Sleap M, Warburton P.** *Physical activity patterns of primary schoolchildren: an interim report.* London, Health Education Authority, 1990.

103. **James WPT.** A public health approach to the problem of obesity. *International Journal of Obesity and Related Metabolic Disorders*, 1995, **19**(Suppl. 3):37S–45S.

104. **Dwyer T et al.** An investigation of the effects of daily physical activity on the health of primary school students in South Australia. *International Journal of Epidemiology*, 1983, **12**:308–313.

105. **Worsley A, Coonan W, Worsley A.** The first body owner's programme: an integrated school-based physical and nutrition programme. *Health Promotion*, 1987, **2**:39–49.

106. **Rajan U.** Management of childhood obesity — Singapore perspective. In: Ismael MN, ed. *Proceedings of the First Scientific Meeting on Obesity.* Kuala Lumpur, Malaysian Society for the Study of Obesity (MASSO), 1996, **1**:131–137.

107. **Davis K, Christoffel KK.** Obesity in preschool and school-age children. Treatment early and often is best. *Archives of Pediatric and Adolescent Medicine*, 1994, **148**:1257–1261.

108. **Leung AK, Robson WL.** Childhood obesity. *Postgraduate Medicine*, 1990, **87**:123–130.

PART V

Challenges for the new millennium

11. Conclusions and recommendations

11.1 General conclusions

1. Obesity (BMI ≥30) is a disease that is largely preventable through lifestyle changes. Overweight (BMI ≥25) is a major determinant of many other NCDs including NIDDM, CHD and stroke, and increases the risk of several types of cancer, gallbladder disease, musculoskeletal disorders and respiratory symptoms. In some populations, the metabolic consequences of weight gain start at modest levels of overweight. The costs attributable to obesity are high not only in terms of premature death and health care but also in terms of disability and a diminished quality of life.

2. The prevalence of overweight and obesity is rapidly increasing worldwide. In many developing countries overweight and obesity coexist with undernutrition. This constitutes a double burden for these countries, and their efforts to combat both should be carefully balanced. There is an urgent need to prevent or reverse unhealthy trends in diet and physical activity patterns in developing countries.

3. Some individuals may become overweight and obese because they have a genetic or biological predisposition to gain weight readily in an unfavourable environment. However, the fundamental causes of the obesity epidemic are societal, resulting from an environment that promotes sedentary lifestyles and the consumption of high-fat, energy-dense diets. These two principal factors interact so that, while it is possible for people who sustain moderately high levels of physical activity throughout life to tolerate diets with a higher fat content (e.g. 30–40% of energy), increasing evidence suggests that lower fat intakes (e.g. 20–25% of energy) are needed to minimize energy imbalance and weight gain in sedentary individuals and societies.

4. Prevention of overweight and obesity should begin early in life, and should involve the development and maintenance of lifelong healthy eating and physical activity patterns. In adults, the prevention of overweight should include efforts to prevent further weight gain even when BMI is still in the acceptable range. Healthy lifestyles, combining balanced diets of lower energy density (increased amounts of vegetables, fruits, grains and cereals) with increased levels of physical activity (such as walking) and reductions in sedentary behaviour, should be promoted. Prevention is not just the responsibility of individuals but also requires structural changes in societies.

5. The management of individuals who are already obese should combine a primary goal of long-term weight maintenance with appropriate treatment to achieve a modest weight loss (5–15% of initial weight) and the management of comorbidities. Individuals and groups at high risk of becoming obese in the future because they are overweight (BMI 25–29.9) should also receive medical attention but here the emphasis should be on prevention of weight gain. Appropriate support and assistance for making sustainable dietary, physical, activity and other healthy lifestyle changes should be an intrinsic part of all management strategies. Drug therapy and surgery can be considered as adjuvant therapy for obese individuals who fail to respond to primary management approaches, especially when there is concurrent risk from other NCDs. However, many countries lack health care delivery systems to implement such a management system. There is an urgent need for adequate training of health professionals and selected lay people, based on the principles outlined above and recognizing that stigmatization of the obese is counterproductive.

6. Obesity cannot be prevented or managed solely at the individual level. Communities, governments, the media and the food industry need to work together to modify the environment so that it is less conducive to weight gain. Such partnerships are required to ensure that effective and sustainable changes in diet and everyday levels of physical activity can be achieved throughout the community. This approach will also allow obesity prevention and management strategies to be harmonized with existing public health policies and programmes for the control of all NCDs.

11.2 Recommendations

The recommendations in sections 11.2.1–11.2.3 are mainly concerned with identifying priority areas for further research, while those in section 11.2.4 deal primarily with the strategies and actions required for the effective management of the global epidemic of obesity.

11.2.1 Defining the problem of overweight and obesity

International classification of overweight and obesity

1. General recommendations

To ensure that meaningful comparisons between populations can be made, the classification of overweight and obesity should be standardized on an international basis, as follows:

- *Adults*. The existing WHO classification of adult body weight status based on BMI should be used with minor modifications. The category of "overweight" (BMI ≥25) should be subdivided into "preobese" (BMI 25–29.9) and "obese" (BMI ≥30). The category of obese should be further subdivided into the following three classes:

— Obese class I: BMI 30–34.9;
— Obese class II: BMI 35–39.9;
— Obese class III: BMI ≥40.

- *Children*. The existing WHO classification of overweight and obesity in children based on weight-for-height values of +2SD or more of the median NCHS (National Center for Health Statistics) reference curves should be used until a new consensus is reached and a more appropriate classification system can be recommended. Caution is needed when interpreting BMI data collected from populations with stunted children, especially in countries undergoing a rapid nutrition transition, as the relationship of BMI to adiposity may be altered.

2. *Priority areas for further research*

Priority should be given to research on:

- The establishment of the most useful standard method of defining childhood and adolescent obesity, which should then be used to formulate new reference curves for growth and to evaluate existing and future child and adolescent data from around the world.

- The validity and tracking of simple measures of excess weight, e.g. BMI-for-age and sex in children and adolescents from different societies and ethnic groups.

- The relationship between BMI and adiposity in stunted children.

- BMI standards for the elderly (>60 years or >80 years).

International comparisons of obesity rates

3. *General recommendations*

Cross-sectional studies of nationally representative samples should be regularly undertaken in all WHO regions to facilitate international comparisons of adulthood obesity rates, to predict the magnitude of the future obesity problem, and to monitor and evaluate the effectiveness of intervention strategies. These studies should document BMI and waist circumference and assess progressively the variety of intervention strategies under way. In particular:

- Countries in the WHO African Region, Region of the Americas, South-East Asia and Eastern Mediterranean Regions should give priority to regular larger-scale surveys of body weight status.

- Data should be recorded according to a standard protocol, i.e. using the WHO classification system for body weight status (BMI ≥25 for overweight and BMI ≥30 for obesity), and based on measured rather than self-reported height and weight.

- Data should be age-standardized and divided according to urban and rural areas.

- Where appropriate, data should be linked to morbidity and mortality outcomes classified, for example, in accordance with ICD-10.[1]

- Countries with the highest obesity rates and/or with rapidly rising secular trends in obesity should be identified within each WHO region and highlighted in regional reports.

- Waist circumference measurements should be included as a useful additional tool for more readily identifying NCD risk.

11.2.2 *Establishing the true costs of the problem of overweight and obesity*

Health impact of overweight and obesity in adults

1. General recommendations

The health consequences of overweight and obesity should be fully evaluated in all parts of the world and among different ethnic groups, as follows:

- While short-duration studies are useful for identifying the major health impact of obesity, long-term monitoring of health indicators should be carried out to determine the full range and impact of obesity-related illnesses, and where the outcome (e.g. cancer) is the result of a multistage process in which obesity has an effect on some, but not necessarily all, stages.

- Standard procedures for estimating the relative risks of chronic health problems associated with weight gain and obesity should be established.

- The prevalence and relative risks in different societies of the chronic health problems associated with obesity should be documented.

- The psychosocial impact of weight gain should be re-evaluated using modern psychosocial techniques.

2. Priority areas for further research

Priority should be given to research on:

---

[1] *International Statistical Classification of Diseases and Related Health Problems. Tenth Revision. Vol. 1. Tabular list.* Geneva, World Health Organization, 1992.

- The relationship between obesity and the development of certain cancers.

- The non-fatal health consequences associated with obesity, especially in developing countries.

- The interactions between measures of fatness (specifically BMI and waist circumference) and both dietary factors and physical activity in determining obesity comorbidities.

- The sex- and population-specific relationships between measures of fatness (specifically BMI and waist circumference) and both morbidity and mortality.

Health impact of overweight and obesity in childhood

3. General recommendations

The health consequences associated with overweight and obesity in childhood and adolescence should be investigated further.

4. Priority areas for further research

Priority should be given to research on:

- The long-term health consequences of childhood obesity and its persistence into adulthood.

- The implications of early excess weight gain in different populations and ethnic groups.

- The nature of the association between rapid childhood growth, early menarche and the later risk of breast cancer.

Health impact of weight loss

5. General recommendations

The health benefits and risks of weight loss should be further investigated through well controlled studies that distinguish between unintentional weight loss (which may result from underlying disease or smoking) and intentional weight loss.

6. Priority areas for further research

Priority should be given to research on:

- An accurate definition of the health benefits and risks for both morbidity and mortality of sustained weight loss (i.e. for more than 2 and preferably 5 years).

- The quantification of the health impact of varying degrees of weight loss in individuals, with and without coexisting disease.

- The impact of weight cycling on obesity-associated illness and the likelihood of future weight gain.

- The impact on intentional weight loss of alterations in the diet and physical activity.

Economic impact of overweight and obesity

7. General recommendations

The economic burden of overweight and obesity should be systematically evaluated in all regions of the world using a standardized methodology. For this reason:

- A variety of health care systems should be evaluated so that different countries and regions can apply the analyses to their own national and regional policies.

- Wherever possible, assessments should include an analysis of the broader social and quality of life issues relating to excess weight gain.

8. Priority area for further research

Priority should be given to research on:

- The evaluation of the relative cost-effectiveness of different management strategies aimed at both the prevention and treatment of excess weight gain.

11.2.3 Understanding how the problem of overweight and obesity develops

Providing a basis for intervention strategies

1. General recommendations

To enable the global problem of obesity to be tackled in a coherent and progressive manner, it is essential that the range of factors implicated in its development, from both an individual and a population perspective, should be fully characterized and investigated through a coherent strategy of short- and long-term studies. In particular, the relative importance of dietary factors and physical activity patterns associated with a modern lifestyle should be investigated further.

2. Priority areas for further research

Priority should be given to research on:

- Dietary factors, including:

    — the influence of the energy density and/or fat content of the diet on the propensity to consume excess energy relative to requirement, and how this relationship is influenced by different levels of physical activity;

— the quantitative significance of sweetened foods or sweet–fat combination foods in promoting a passive overconsumption of energy;

— how taste preferences and eating patterns (including those associated with the consumption of energy-dense diets) develop during childhood and whether these are associated with any specific developmental stages;

— the optimum ranges of energy density and nutrient/energy ratios for children's diets that will promote appropriate growth and development but prevent the development of excess adiposity.

• Physical activity patterns, including:

— the relationship between levels of physical activity and future weight gain;

— factors that promote and reinforce physical inactivity;

— the relationship between obesity and sedentary behaviours such as television viewing, video games and computer work in a wide variety of countries;

— quantification of the amount of voluntary energy expenditure necessary to prevent weight gain in adults in sedentary occupations;

— changes in food selection in the general population with relatively small changes in levels of physical activity.

• Societal and cultural factors influencing energy intake and physical activity patterns, including:

— the effects on the development of overweight and obesity in children of existing programmes to combat undernutrition in developing countries;

— the relative influence of different aspects of modernization on the energy density of the food supply and levels of physical activity;

— the influence of socioeconomic status, including educational level, on the risk of becoming obese;

— the process of nutrition transition and its impact on average body weight in a population.

• Genetic/biological factors involved in weight gain and obesity, including:

— the identification of genes and mutations responsible for the susceptibility of some individuals and groups of people to weight gain in conjunction with an energy-dense diet and a sedentary mode of life;

— the relative importance of vulnerable periods of life for the development of obesity.

11.2.4 *Addressing the problem of overweight and obesity*

Focus on prevention strategies

1. General recommendations

Considerably more attention should be given to strategies aimed at preventing weight gain and obesity, since these are likely to be more cost-effective and have a greater positive impact on the long-term control of body weight than those designed to deal with obesity once it has fully developed. In particular:

- Action should be taken at the following three levels to develop effective strategies for the prevention of overweight and obesity:
  - *universal/public health prevention* (directed at everyone in the population);
  - *selective prevention* (directed at subgroups of the population with an above-average risk of developing obesity);
  - *targeted prevention* (directed at high-risk individuals with existing weight problems but who are not yet obese).

- Small-scale pilot projects should be carried out to determine the practicality and appropriateness of specific intervention strategies.

- Practical evaluation of obesity-prevention programmes should be based on the assessment of changes in the prevalence of overweight (BMI >25) combined with short-term process indicators of dietary change and physical activity levels. Assessment of changes in the prevalence of obesity (BMI >30) and its comorbidities is less reliable but may be useful in the long term. Changes in the incidence of obesity and mean population BMI are more accurate measures of change in population weight status that can be used for a more detailed and closely controlled analysis.

- Current obesity-prevention initiatives should be evaluated, their limitations identified and their designs improved.

Improving physical activity levels and healthy eating

2. General recommendations

Prevention of overweight and obesity should begin early in life, and should be based on the development and maintenance of lifelong healthy eating and physical activity patterns. In particular:

- Schools should promote physical activity by incorporating a variety of recreational activities into teaching curricula. They should also encourage healthy eating through training in practical food skills and by adopting healthy nutrition standards for school meals.

- Community facilities should be designed and traffic and town planning policies developed to facilitate everyday walking and exercise in adults and children.

- Workplaces should promote physical activity and healthy eating by providing exercise and changing facilities, adopting healthy nutrition catering standards, and initiating other appropriate schemes.

- Interventions aimed at the prevention and management of obesity should be carefully designed so that they do not cause undue fear of fatness and precipitate eating disorders.

- Consumers should be educated and encouraged to demand food products of high nutritional quality.

- The strategies adopted should be population-specific, especially with respect to economic circumstances. Thus, for example, the main aim of physical activity interventions in developing countries should be to prevent the decline in such activity that usually accompanies economic development, whereas the main emphasis in affluent societies should be on discouraging existing patterns of sedentary behaviour.

Need for public health strategies
Population-based (universal) public health strategies should be adopted that aim to reduce the obesity-promoting aspects of the environment and to improve a population's knowledge of obesity and its management. In particular:

- Strategies should be multisectoral; governments, regional authorities, the food industry, the media, communities and the consumer should all be engaged in collaborative programmes.

- Strategies should aim to produce an environment that supports improved eating and physical activity habits throughout the entire community.

- Novel and practical strategies that go beyond traditional health promotion programmes should be investigated.

- Strategies should aim to achieve the optimum population median BMI range of 21–23. Adults in developing countries are likely to gain greater benefit from a median BMI of 23, whereas adults in affluent societies with a more sedentary lifestyle are likely to gain greater benefit from a median BMI of 21.

- Strategies should be adapted to the specific characteristics of each community or country.
- Improving the standard of living of all sectors of society, and especially of often neglected native or minority populations, should be a priority for public health action in developing and newly industrialized countries.
- Lessons learned from past campaigns on other public health problems (e.g. poor immunization rates and drink-driving) should be carefully considered and incorporated when designing public health strategies for controlling obesity.

Need for health care and community services

3. General recommendations

Obesity-management programmes should be established within health care and community services to target individuals and subgroups of the population who have developed, or are at risk of developing, obesity and its comorbidities. In particular:

- Primary health care services should play the dominant role, but hospital and specialist services are also required to deal with very high-risk individuals.
- Steps should be taken to ensure the clear communication between the different levels of health care service that is essential.
- Weight-management services and protocols should be based on the principles outlined in this report but should be adapted to the circumstances of each country.
- In addition to strategies aimed at modest weight loss, strategies for weight maintenance and management of obesity comorbidities should be an integral part of management programmes for individuals with existing overweight and obesity.
- Simple anthropometric methods, e.g. waist circumference and waist:hip ratio, should be used to identify overweight individuals at increased risk of obesity-related illness due to abdominal fat accumulation.
- The efficacy of management schemes should be evaluated over a period of at least 1 year and preferably 2–5 years.

4. Priority area for further research

Priority should be given to:

- Further investigation to determine whether documented successful management programmes for overweight in children and adolescents can be replicated in different situations and in different populations.

Improved training in the management of obesity

5. General recommendations

The training of all health care workers involved in the management of obese patients should urgently be improved. In particular:

- Obesity should be viewed as a serious medical condition in its own right; it is a disease that can be treated with lifestyle modification and effective management. Obesity should be treated even when comorbidities are not present.

- Negative attitudes of health care professionals towards obesity and obese patients should be overcome, since the stigmatization of obese individuals adds to the existing burden of this disease.

Need for evaluation

6. General recommendations

Systematic assessment and evaluation should be a routine part of all interventions aimed at preventing and managing overweight and obesity. In particular:

- The effectiveness of different weight-management therapies should be evaluated in clearly defined groups of patients and in the social context of each country.

- The effectiveness of all public health programmes aimed at preventing weight gain in the population should be evaluated.

- Sound experimental design and statistical principles should be used to critically evaluate the impact of each proposed intervention.

7. Priority area for further research

Priority should be given to:

- Further long-term studies to evaluate the risk–benefit ratio of prolonged and integrated management schemes (with and without the use of drugs) for weight loss and maintenance in terms of mortality, comorbidities, quality of life and cost-effectiveness.

Shared responsibility
Since obesity cannot be prevented or managed solely at the individual level, governments, the food industry, international agencies, the media, communities and individuals should all work together to modify the environment so that it is less conducive to weight gain. In particular:

- Steps should be taken to ensure the synergistic interaction of national policies on nutrition and the control of NCDs in the prevention and management of overweight, obesity and associated comorbidities.

- The activities of the health, educational and agricultural sectors should be coordinated to ensure effective government action for the prevention and management of overweight.

- Strategies for integrated approaches to the prevention and management of overweight should include consumer education, the development and implementation of dietary guidelines, food labelling, nutrition and physical education in schools, altered feeding programmes, and efforts to ensure truth in advertising.

- The food industry should be responsible for developing and promoting affordable healthy food products.

- Governments should enforce adherence to regulations governing the marketing, advertising and labelling of food.

- The media should not induce or exacerbate eating disorders in societies where they do not exist or encourage the stigmatization of the obese in societies where this is unknown.

- The support of international agencies and nongovernmental organizations dealing with NCDs other than obesity should be sought, since this is essential for developing successful public health efforts to control obesity in developing and newly industrialized countries.

Acknowledgements

The Consultation expressed deep appreciation to the International Obesity Task Force (IOTF) chaired by Professor W.P.T. James of the Rowett Research Institute (Aberdeen, Scotland) who was instrumental in the preparation and convening of the Consultation. The Consultation also thanked the authors of the background documents for the Consultation: Professor P. Björntorp, University of Gothenburg, Gothenburg, Sweden; Professor G.A. Bray, Louisiana State University, Baton Rouge, LA, USA; Dr K.K. Carroll, University of Western Ontario, London, Ontario, Canada; Dr A. Chuchalin, Pulmonology Research Institute, Moscow, Russian Federation; Dr W.H. Dietz, New England Medical Center, Boston, MA, USA; Dr G.E. Ehrlich, University of Pennsylvania, Philadelphia, PA, USA; Dr J.O. Hill, University of Colorado, Denver, CO, USA; Dr F.X. Pi-Sunyer, St. Luke's Roosevelt Hospital Center and Columbia University, New York, NY, USA; Dr W.H.M. Saris, University of Maastricht, Maastricht, Netherlands; Dr J.C. Seidell, National Institute of Public Health and the Environment, Bilthoven, Netherlands; Professor P. Zimmet and colleagues, International Diabetes Institute, Caulfield, Victoria, Australia.

The Consultation also recognized the valuable contributions made by the following individuals who provided comments on the background documents: Professor R.L. Atkinson, University of Wisconsin, Madison, WI, USA; Professor H.W. Blackburn, University of Minnesota, Minneapolis, MN, USA; Dr K. Ge, Institute of Nutrition and Food Hygiene, Chinese Academy of Preventive Medicine, Beijing, China; Professor A. Kissebah, Medical College of Wisconsin, Milwaukee, WI, USA; Dr A. Kurpad, St Johns Medical College, Bangalore, India; Professor J. Mann, University of Otago, Dunedin, New Zealand; Professor K. Norum, University of Oslo, Oslo, Norway; Dr A. Prentice, Dunn Clinical Nutrition Centre, Cambridge, England; Professor S. Rössner, Karolinska Hospital, Stockholm, Sweden; Professor P.S. Shetty, London School of Hygiene and Tropical Medicine, London, England; Dr L. Sjöstrom, Gothenburg University, Gothenburg, Sweden; Professor T.I.A. Sörensen, Copenhagen Municipality Hospital, Copenhagen, Denmark; Dr K. Steyn, Chronic Diseases of Lifestyle, Tygerber, South Africa; Professor M. Wahlqvist, Monash Medical Centre, Clayton, Victoria, Australia; Dr R. Weinsier, University of Alabama, Birmingham, AL, USA; Dr D.F. Williamson, Centers for Disease Control and Alabama, Birmingham, AL, USA; Dr D.F. Williamson, Centers for Disease Control and Prevention, Atlanta, GA, USA; Dr R. Wing, Western Psychiatric Institute and Clinics, Pittsburgh, PA, USA. In addition, the Consultation expressed its gratitude to the following nongovernmental organizations, which also reviewed the background documents and provided valuable comments: International Association for Adolescent Health; International Diabetes Federation; International Life Sciences Institute. Comments were also kindly provided by the South African Society for Obesity and the World Sugar Research Organization.

Special acknowledgement was made by the Consultation to the IOTF secretariat members Dr T. Gill and Ms V. Lakin for the time they spent in preparing for the Consultation and finalizing the report.

The Consultation expressed special appreciation to Dr S. Dehler, Ms R. Imperial and Mrs P. Robertson of the Programme of Nutrition, World Health Organization, Geneva, Switzerland, for their efforts in preparing for the Consultation and in revising and formatting the report, and to Mr J. Akré, also of WHO, and Mr J. Bland for their editorial assistance.

Annex
Criteria for evaluating commercial institutions involved in weight loss[1]

Appropriate criteria for evaluating commercial institutions involved in weight loss should include:

1. Identification and recording of an individual's BMI or an equivalent weight-for-height before advice is given.
2. Methods of record-keeping and analysis open to scrutiny by a health centre if patients are to be referred from the centre. Data on the health centre's patients should be available on request.
3. Use of an admission protocol that excludes those within the desirable weight range from a weight-reduction programme.
4. Identification of an individual or family-based approach to weight reduction.
5. Provision of clear written as well as oral guidance on the dietary regimen, used together with details of the expert(s) used in drawing up such guidance.
6. Specification of the methods used, if any, for encouraging physical activity.
7. Definition of the nature of behavioural modification programmes, the frequency of visits, the use of group or individual support and the origin of the behavioural scheme.
8. Whether food additives, drugs or other medicaments (e.g. ephedrine, caffeine homoeopathic remedies, and nutrient supplements) are used in association with therapy.
9. Methods for verifying therapeutic claims made in advertisements or in weight-management programmes.
10. The methods chosen to alert the members' doctors to untoward effects.
11. Any plans for coordinated activity with a health centre on weight management.
12. The experience, training and qualifications of staff.
13. The success criteria offered to clients.

---

[1] Adapted, with the permission of the publisher, from *Obesity in Scotland. A rational clinical guideline recommended for use in Scotland*. Edinburgh, Scottish Intercollegiate Guidelines Network, 1996.

www.ingramcontent.com/pod-product-compliance
Lightning Source LLC
Chambersburg PA
CBHW081531120626
46550CB00009B/2684